DIAGNOSING
DEMONS
AN INTRODUCTION TO MENTAL ILLNESS
AND SPIRITUAL WARFARE

MINISTER ANTONIO C. ANDERSON MS, MSW

CLAY BRIDGES
PRESS

Diagnosing Demons

An Introduction to Mental Illness and Spiritual Warfare

Copyright © 2021 by Minister Antonio C. Anderson MS, MSW

Published by Clay Bridges in Houston, TX
www.claybridgespress.com

Scripture quotations are taken from the New King James Version®. Copyright © 1982 by Thomas Nelson. Used by permission. All rights reserved.

ISBN 978-1-953300-68-3 (paperback)
ISBN 978-1-953300-67-6 (ebook)

Special Sales: Most Clay Bridges titles are available in special quantity discounts. Custom imprinting or excerpting can also be done to fit special needs. For standard bulk orders, go to www.claybridgesbulk.com. For specialty press or large orders, contact Clay Bridges at info@claybridgespress.com.

I dedicate this book to God, without whom nothing in mental health, spiritual warfare, or anything else would ever matter.

I dedicate this to my mother, Apostle Jenni'fer, who instilled God in me and exhibited a relationship with Christ so strong that psychology, philosophy, social work, and many other professors could not kill my relationship with Christ.

To the queen of my heart, Adriana Anderson, who believes in us so much that my only option is to improve in life.

To my courageous son, Kareem, who teaches me how to raise a giant.

To my daughter, Ariel, who teaches me how to love a princess.

Finally, to anyone struggling to make sense out of thoughts and behaviors that fail to make sense.

You matter!

TABLE OF CONTENTS

SPECIAL THANKS

I would like to thank my father, Tony Anderson Sr.; my brothers, Thor Anderson and Leandrew Chapman; and my sisters, Love Ralph, Joy Banks-Chapman, and Kat Anderson.

I would like to thank "The Squad from God," Lead Pastor Jay Haizlip, Pastor Johnny Thompson, Deacon Javier Amador, Deacon Marvin Torres, Deacon Eddie Camacho, Deacon Anthony Martinez, Deacon Bob, Deacon Frank "Unreal" Meza, and all the incredible members of the Dream Team and the Sanctuary Church of Costa Mesa for being the type of church that facilitates masterpieces out of broken vessels. I would like to thank Pastor Jeff Ludington, lead pastor of Generations Church, who will forever be family to me in this life and the next. He exudes a genuine love for people and God that has become rare in far too many churches. I would like to thank Pastor Brad Carter of Calvary Church in North Carolina. Pastor Carter, people make statues of men like you. You are a giant! Robert Hotchkin of Men on the Frontlines, that Southern California Man camp was so high in Christ that we never came down! It's not about time; it's simply time! My entire being changed, so I thank you for your yes to His will! I would like to thank my brothers in the trenches, Keith Herr, Sam Hubinette, and Jeremiah Cortez, As Iron Sharpens Iron for Life Men. I would like to thank all the staff of Lucid Books for taking my project. I would like to thank Casey Cease, CEO of Lucid Books, for taking my call just to motivate me while he was on vacation. Thank you to Megan Poling, Director of Author Relations, who spoke to me like I was an old friend of hers and really blessed the process before it even began. I would like to thank Laurie Waller, the

Director of Writing and Editing Services at Lucid Books, who was straightforward about my book and showed me its strengths. Alisa DeMarco, Marketing at Lucid Books, thank you for spending so much time explaining the strategies and marketing knowledge for this project. Sarah Ray, Publishing Coordinator at Lucid Books, thank you for strategically putting everything in place for a painless project.

FOREWORD

Nature is filled with animals and species that have the incredible ability to camouflage themselves in various atmospheres so their original nature can be hidden, remaining unseen and unrecognized while living right before our eyes in plain sight.

Can this be true of mental illness?

Can the true nature of a mental condition be camouflaged in an environment, hidden behind the atmosphere of clinical names, medical terminology, and study settings and sessions that may often deny its true original nature?

Antonio Anderson's work will explore those very questions and more. Get ready to be introduced to secular intellectual scholarship and powerful biblical events that are educational, thought-provoking, informative, inspirational, and life-changing.

This book is an honest and careful exploration of both clinical and biblical case studies of how Jesus Christ approached the appearance of the many mental moments and encounters with life-changing power. It demonstrates how we approach and attempt to analytically address many mental disorders with the greatest of intention and in the best efforts of our human abilities.

This work will begin to introduce us to the many ways Jesus the Messiah managed what we may call or perceive to be mental illness and how His heart, life, and words were powerful and intentionally confrontational to remedy, recognize, and resolve issues that were rooted demonically in origin and how He actively addressed the true nature of what He experienced with authoritative power. His Word became the solution of peace, healing, and total deliverance for the total person—mind, body, and soul.

My dear friend and brother Antonio has devoted many years of time and study to bridge the clinical and Christ-producing volume of work that will inspire, enlighten, and educate those who have been given the challenge of daring to understand biblical truth and live devoted to the challenge of having the problem in one hand and the solution in the other while being committed to bridging the two. I consider this work to be a Master's piece.

—Johnny Thompson, Pastor

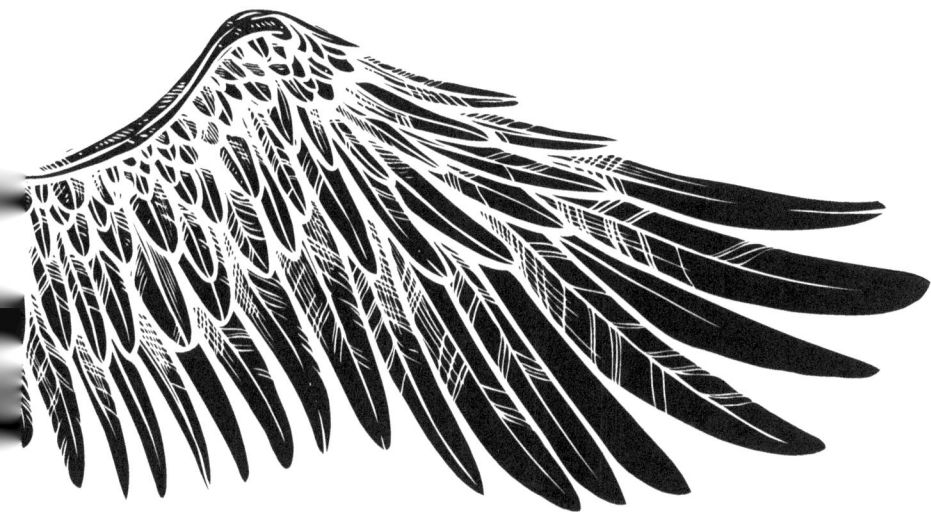

INTRODUCTION

Diagnosing Demons is a book to be found on the shelf of every mental health professional, pastor, and spiritual leader.

There is a thin line between psychosis and demonology. The DSM5 defines psychosis as "a mental health problem that causes people to perceive or interpret things differently from those around them. This might involve hallucinations or delusions." Wikipedia defines demonology as "the study of demons or beliefs about demons, and the hierarchy of demons. They may be nonhuman, separable souls, or discarnate spirits which have never inhabited a body." When delusions and demons are defined from a spiritual realm, we are looking at the client who is experiencing or seeing things in the spiritual realm. *Diagnosing Demons* gives an in-depth look into those experiences.

Antonio Anderson used wisdom in preparing you, the reader, for the time you will spend reading this book. Satan is cunning and strategic; he will retaliate against you for every knowledge you gain against him. The Scripture states, "Lest Satan should get an advantage of us: for we are not ignorant of his devices" (2 Cor. 2:11, KJV). The author has stated, "So many on my team have prayed for you while you read this, for the captivity of every thought." "Casting down imaginations, and every high thing that exalteth itself against the knowledge of God, and bringing into captivity every thought to the obedience of Christ" (2 Cor. 10:5, KJV).

Since 1979, God has used me to deliver many from demon possession. From the first deliverance to today and after years of studying psychology, I have come to understand that mental disorders and demon possession are very closely related. The symptoms are similar, but the treatment is never the same. For years I avoided studying psychology because I felt it was a direct conflict with the Spirit of God. Fast-forward to now, and I had to relinquish my beliefs of psychology and my humanitarian theories that most people have, including those working in the field, about mental disorder.

This book helps clear up misconceptions, clearly defining the difference and the problematic role a therapist, pastor, or leader has when counseling someone who may be demon possessed, oppressed, or tormented, or someone who feels they are inhabited by a demon when there may be a valid chemical imbalance or personality disorder.

This is spiritual warfare!

Diagnosing Demons introduces the origin of Satan and the warfare between psychology and the satanic realm. Anderson indicates that the bite of the fruit brought power to Satan's kingdom. This started a revolt against mankind, the humanity God created out of His unconditional love. Defeating the plans and schemes of the strong man is a war we must all face in our day-to-day existence. This book is intended to create awareness of the warfare in the world and is not inclusive of mental illness. Satan comes to kill, steal, and destroy. Mental illness and personality disorders are also destroyers of families, homes, lives, and individuals.

This book helps bring into perspective the destroyer qualities of both Satan and mental illness. Anderson states, "At that very moment, the fact that Adam and Eve looked for leaves to cover themselves because they were naked meant that anxiety, shame, guilt, depression, and insecurity—all of that happened in the mind—were an introduction to mental illness by Satan who came to kill, steal, and destroy. Not only were they now dealing with a bombardment of negative emotions they had never experienced, but they were also kicked out of the only home they had known."

Until we as the children of God understand we are warriors for Christ in a battle on this earth, we will continue to lose many battles. We need to understand the strategies of Satan. Every mental illness does not have a satanic root. And every personality disorder cannot be treated with medication. It is only the wisdom from God that will give us the discernment to know the difference. What does Jesus do to defeat demonic spirits? While you are reading this book, think about how you would respond. Anderson leaves his readers with a challenge: "If a possessed man walked into your church, how would he be received? Would he be pushed out, or would he be surrounded by a deliverance church of prayer warriors? If it is not the latter, are you in the church Jesus imagined? Jesus laid hands on and delivered many people just like this man."

"All mental illness can be battled."

"There is nothing new under the sun."

I pray you enjoy reading this book as much as I have. Mostly, you will have gained insight to not be ignorant of Satan's devices.

May these words be etched upon your heart: "Now thanks be unto God, which always causeth us to triumph in Christ, and maketh manifest the savour of his knowledge by us in every place" (2 Cor. 2:14, KJV).

Blessing, Honor, and His Love,
Dr. JJMB Chapman, Beyond the Walls Ministries
Worship & Deliverance Center International

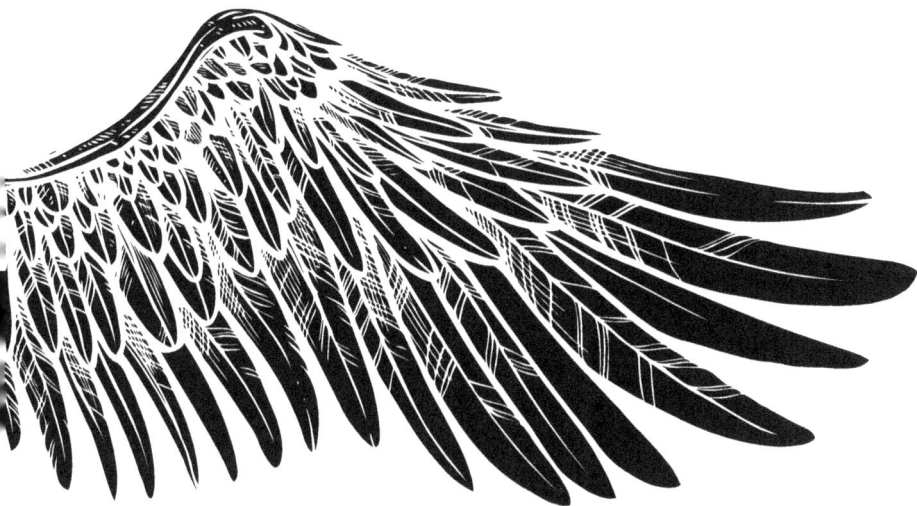

CHAPTER 1

THE SADDEST BEAUTY—THE FIRST IMPRESSION

These things I have spoken to you, so that in Me you may have peace. In the world you will have tribulation; but be of good cheer, I have overcome the world.

—John 16:33

It was an overcast morning in 1990, typical for a summer-morning drive through the San Francisco Bay Area. We lived in San Jose at the time and were traveling to Treasure Island in San Francisco, California. The type of dense fog we faced that day never seemed to make it to the "Welcome to San Francisco!" brochure. I cannot imagine the photo befitting this postcard trolley ride while visitors gripped for dear life into the unknown mist. As in life, some truths must be experienced in order to be disappointed by reality. That day had one of those "hellafied" luminous skies in the middle of the day watching seagulls plot to steal fish lunches from oblivious tourists.

This day was another olfactory-violating experience of what looked like a hundred obese seals fighting over two feet of space like Alcatraz prisoners at the commissary. People watched them, amazed; I watched people, perplexed at their amazement. This experience was a blatant disrespect to my appetite for "The World's Best Clam Chowder," a title every seafood restaurant for the next five blocks apparently held. You don't have to be a sheep, but then again, when in Rome, they say. After trying two bests while holding my nose, I had to make another hard choice. Shall I walk up two miles at an 80-degree angle to Ghiradelli Square for overpriced ice cream and richly sweetened lattes? Or shall I try the dusty wax museum or an obsolete, underwhelming who-cares-anyway record? I am not bitter; I just hate double-fisted memories of vanilla tourist traps. Before you leave, you do have the right book. We are going to get to the good stuff, but let me set the backstory of why mental health or spiritual warfare even matters to me.

On that day, absolutely nothing could have diminished the enthusiastic anxiety shared by my friend Michael and me as we sat behind captain seats, scrunched on a bench in the back of a luxury old-school van that Paul, Mike's father, owned. It looked exactly like 1990. It was dark brown on the exterior with golden glitter swirls and two-tinted oval concave windows on the rear sides that looked like two fishbowl halves. The interior was a premeditated Moulin Rouge like a mobile speakeasy.

Michael and I were both 10 years old, and we were grown men. We made a pact that it was the last evening we would answer to being called kids. Twenty-four hours from that morning, we would be donning navy blues, freshly bald, and *men*. We were fully engulfed in boot camp for the Naval Sea Cadet Academy hosted by Treasure Island, or what we pre-shipmen would call "hell on water." We did not know what we were getting into since our previous experiences to this point were spending four to eight hours performing drills bimonthly. Now was the real divider of heroes thrust into a full two weeks of 24/7 boot camp.

Since we had no idea what to expect, we were cursed with having two survivors, Mike's older brothers, David and Paul, who had both spent at least three summers at boot camp. Paul, who was 18, was about to enlist as a first class petty officer in the real navy. Paul was our go-to on all things manly. David, who was younger than Paul by two years, loathed that Paul was given so much credit for just being 18 and able to join the military. David had tortured us on our trip, despising that we had focused on Paul rather than his personal experiences and advice.

The boys' mother, Dianne, insisted that David and Paul allow us to have our own experience and not haunt us. David saw haunting as a great plan. He told us that on the first night, we would be fit with catheters because there were no bathrooms. He also told us that if we talked back in any way, we would be beaten with rock-filled socks at night by the staff. We were trying to play it tough, but I recall reminding myself to blink and found it hard to swallow. My pupils were wide enough to see through the blackout curtains gracing the van. Michael and I were side by side. We did not even have eye contact as we tried to adhere to our newfound manliness.

Before we made it to Treasure Island, we passed through downtown San Francisco right when the sun was retiring, beckoning his coming bride, the smoldering moon. The biggest impact I would face was only moments away but would immediately unleash a greater purpose within me. I liked walking the Golden Gate Bridge. I always leaned over the edge, peered at the treacherous, uninviting, dirty-looking, choppy, brown water, and wondered how anyone could be so depressed that they would jump into it. I guess that was the point. I was blissfully ignorant to what it was like to want to take my life. I literally climbed those steel ropes that looked like they were created by King Kong's hands and thought to myself, "How can you stand right here on the impossible and not believe anything is possible?"

How can you stand right here on the impossible and not believe anything is possible?

It was at this sensitive juncture that we were grounded by Mike's classy yet elegant-as-a-whiskey-bar-sounding maiden exclaiming, "Would you just look at this (four-legged female dog)? She must be crazy!" Then my mother, Jenni'fer, shielded Mike's and my eyes and told us to stay away from the curtains. That would be the first and last time I would hear those words in a vehicle. My mother went to the front of the van and urged Paul to continue driving. He was at a full stop to witness the spectacle, and it was just the opening that Mike's curiosity needed.

Of course, since it was Mike's vehicle, he did the honors of opening the forbidden curtains, and voilà, there in the middle of a busy downtown street stood a white woman in her mid-to-late 20s. She was beautiful. She had dirty-blond hair and almost eerie lake-blue eyes that were still beautiful even when peering through depressed, bleeding, black eyeliner as she thrust obscenities at willing spectators. She was curvy enough to be in magazines, and she was naked—like not-a-shred-of-clothes naked. I mean Adam-and-Eve-would-not-believe naked. Like just-born, spanked, billed, and thanked by the doctor naked.

After this grand spectacle, there was a decade of silence, or 10 minutes of eternity. Michael and I chuckled and looked at each other, laughing, hoping someone would explain what our insecure, T-shirt-wearing-in-the-pool, self-body-shaming selves could not. Then the same voice that brought us to this point, Dianne's, spoke. "That girl was on some good drugs." And with that, everyone who was not my mother, Mike, or me, laughed and verbally agreed that they solved the case of who they named "Street Sally." At that, the van returned to normal. Maybe drugs meant it was not airborne, so if it was a choice, we could "Just Say No!" like the posters, commercials, T-shirts, shoes, bandanas, and headbands said.

Drugs? thought I. The same drugs that showed a bunch of kids fully clothed standing in a circle with long hair and skateboards on posters all around the world? Could it be that simple? Drugs just explained every behavior that "bizarre" people did, of course, when drugs fit the narrative of what our inexperience and miseducation could not. Yet as ignorant as our response to that experience was, it is not much different than the experiences I came across for decades after that experience throughout the mental health field.

> *If we aim to satisfy our brains with a story and complete the annoyance of the unknown with a plausible explanation, it is all we need to satisfy doing nothing to change the world.*

As I peered out the window, I did not know anything about drugs, but even at the age of 10, I was not sold on drugs being the answer to all unexplainable behaviors. I imagined Street Sally locked eyes with me for a second, and I felt strong empathy for her. I was always the kid with the cape, desperately wanting my chance to save the world. This was even before I understood that being the middle child meant I was a mediator. Now it just means I subconsciously reinforced those middle-child behaviors just because I read something that said I was supposed to, subliminally making those experiences stand out, kind of like the weirdos who take horoscopes seriously. Street Sally—yes, what if she was a victim of an attack and needed to be rescued? She looked sad; she was crying.

This was my first introduction to mental illness. I am still thankful that another tour of the Tenderloin area known for an encampment of thousands of homeless people would not be for another 10 years. Street Sally had shaken me up because I wanted to save this woman, yet salvation seemed beyond my ability to save three UPC labels from the bottom of cereal boxes and wait for a perfect solution to come in the mail. This might have been the single most influential moment that changed everything for me.

If I can be honest with you, as a response to any witnessed response to a stressor, you can be seen by a psychiatrist or psyche team and be given medications and placed on a hold for a diagnosis you may or may not fit. We can blame big pharmaceutical companies, we can blame overzealous psychiatrists, or we can blame the 15 seconds with each patient cookie-cutter diagnosis psychiatrist (yes, we have plenty of those in Orange County) and several other factors. I remember reading about a group of graduate students in a psychology course who self-admitted to a mental health unit based on bogus symptoms and how they were placed on certified holds, prescribed medications, and kept in the facility.

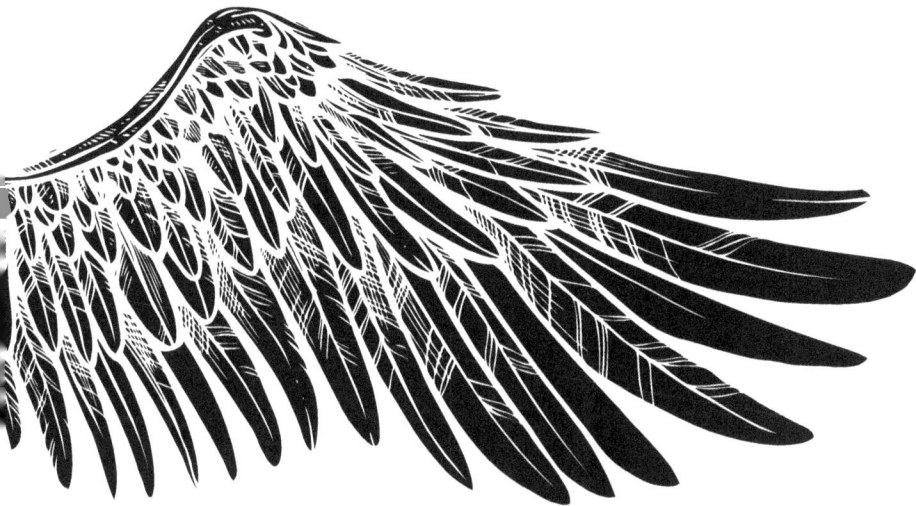

CHAPTER 2

PERFECT BACKDROP TO MENTAL ILLNESS

"Lord, have mercy on my son, for he is an epileptic and suffers severely; for he often falls into the fire and often into the water. So I brought him to Your disciples, but they could not cure him."

Then Jesus answered and said, "O faithless and perverse generation, how long shall I be with you? How long shall I bear with you? Bring him here to Me."

—Matt. 17:14–17

Since we are going to spend the entirety of this book talking about mental health, mental illness, and spiritual warfare, we are going to need a working definition of all three.

1. Mental health is a state of well-being in which the individual realizes his or her own abilities, can cope with the normal stresses of life, can work productively and fruitfully, and is able to contribute to his or her community.

2. Mental illness is a recognized, medically diagnosable illness that results in the significant impairment of an individual's cognitive, affective, or relational abilities. Mental disorders result from biological, developmental, or psychosocial factors and can be managed using approaches comparable to those applied to physical disease (i.e., prevention, diagnosis, treatment, and rehabilitation).

3. Spiritual warfare is a battle against Satan that takes place in the unseen, spiritual dimension and is fought with the weapons that have divine power to demolish strongholds, all while resisting Satan, standing firm in the faith, remaining strong in the Lord, and pursuing the ultimate victory of destroying arguments against the knowledge of God and taking captive every thought to make it obedient to Christ.

I have sat with many church leaders and mental health experts and received many questions about what the purpose of writing this book was. I grew up with a grandfather who was a pastor, two uncles who were pastors, and a mother who is to this day an apostle in Northern California for Beyond the Walls Ministries. The more I learned about psychology growing up, the more I saw the increasing divide between psychology and ultimately a belief in Christ. It came to a point where a professor at California State Long Beach scoffed at me for my belief and stated, "There will be no need for you to go for a doctorate since those degrees are purely left for those in pursuit of becoming godlike themselves." I could not help but laugh as I replayed in my head, "Every knee should bow . . . every tongue should confess that Jesus Christ is Lord" (Phil. 2:10–11).

Leaders in the church asked me how I maintained my strong faith amid learning so much warfare against the church and God in graduate school. Mental health experts either defended their own faith before being interviewed, confused by my questions regarding faith while in a psych ward, or were just annoyed at the implications my line of questioning implored.

I wrote this book because I was prompted by the Holy Spirit to do so. I want you to know this information firsthand early in this book for two reasons.

1. I did not seek to write this book. When the notion came into my mind, the war began. My initial response, though, having earned three master's degrees in general psychology, clinical psychology, and social work and just under 20 years' experience, was that there were far too many more qualified people than me. I felt I was not nearly as knowledgeable or equipped as others to write this book. I tossed and turned on all of it until one day when I was reading the Word I was reminded of the story of Moses and how he was sent to Egypt where he was raised to deliver his people from Pharaoh's hand. It was the same Pharaoh he grew up alongside of like a brother in the very palace where he was raised. Moses did not feel qualified, but God qualified Moses through pruning and obedience. I realized I had the choice to say no, but I did not have the right to say no.

2. If you read this and find yourself understanding the bridge between mental health and spiritual warfare, then you, my brother or sister in Christ, are the reason I wrote this. The completion of this book was an internal "leveling up" for me in my obedience to the will of God

in my life and a pivotal piece of the journey. I do not believe for a second that any book outside of the Holy Bible has the answers to every question. As a matter of fact, I guarantee that this book is not the holy grail of mental health or spiritual warfare by itself. What I do believe is that this book, written on napkins while on vacations, while in other countries, while using the bathroom light past midnight because the idea in my head would not last until daylight, through prayers, through fasting, through more prayers and more fasting, was entirely written from a desire to illustrate God's love for you. No matter what you are going through spiritually or mentally, God is not against you. He is on your side and will see you through (Ps. 118:6).

So many on my team have prayed for you while you read this, for the captivity of every thought in your cognition (2 Cor. 10:5), for restoration of your mind and all that has been taken from you (Joel 2:25), for confirmation within you that you are brand-new in Christ (2 Cor. 5:17), and for assurance that the Lord has plans for your life, plans for welfare and not evil, for a future and hope (Jer. 29:11).

All of that indicates that you do not have this book in your hands by luck or chance. You have this book in your hands as a blessing for your life!

The first case of mental illness began shortly after God created man and woman. In Genesis, we read that Adam had all authority and dominion over everything he encountered in the Garden of Eden, living off the land in his Father's hands. Adam relinquished that authority and dominion the moment he listened to Satan and disobeyed God who had given Adam and Eve clear instructions: "Of every tree of the garden you may freely eat; but of the tree of the knowledge of good and evil you shall not eat, for in the day that you eat of it you shall surely die" (Gen. 2:16–17). Satan in the form of a serpent told them they will not surely die but will become like gods themselves, and so they took a bite of the forbidden fruit.

Biting that fruit gave dominion to Satan. At that very moment, the fact that Adam and Eve looked for leaves to cover themselves because they were naked meant that anxiety, shame, guilt, depression, and insecurity—all of that happened in the mind—were an introduction to mental illness by Satan who came to kill, steal, and destroy. Not only were they now dealing with a bombardment of negative emotions they had never experienced, but they were also kicked out of the only home they had known.

In Luke 8:26–39, we find Jesus healing demon possession. In Gadarenes, opposite Galilee, Jesus steps out of a boat onto land and is met by a demon-possessed man who had been battling demons for a long time. He wore no clothes and lived in tombs. He was bound by shackles and chains and then broke the bonds and was driven into the wilderness by demons. Jesus commanded the unclean spirit to come out of the man and sent the begging demons into the swine that ran into a lake and drowned. The people watching ran to the city to tell others, who returned to find the man in his right mind, sitting at the feet of Jesus.

If you look at the symptoms from a psychological perspective, this man would have had a psyche team evaluate him, strap him to a cold, hard bed, and rush him to the nearest psyche hospital. They would have accepted his insurance and given him a cocktail of meds to "stabilize" him until his behaviors were deemed "normal," or "baseline." Jesus was not afraid of the demons at all. He addressed them by driving them out of the man.

Let's fast-forward.

> *If a possessed man walked into your church, how would he be received? Would he be pushed out, or would he be surrounded by a deliverance church of prayer warriors?*

If it is not the latter, are you in the church Jesus imagined? Jesus laid hands on and delivered many people just like this man.

All mental illness can be battled.

There is nothing new under the sun.

You are not experiencing anything that Jesus did not overcome.

It is covered by His blood.

Some battles are much harder than others. The truth is that anxiety, depression, suicidal ideation, anger, and more are derived from fear. If I get angry with my three-year-old for running in the street, my anger comes from the fear that she will get hit by an oncoming car if she keeps up that behavior.

If I am constantly jumping from the "sparkle" (beginning, sweet stages) of one relationship to another, I sabotage the relationship either subconsciously or consciously due to my insecurities—a fear that I can fall in love with someone and they will end up leaving once they know my flaws. If I fear that I will never get past this emotional battle and that taking my life is the only answer, I am in fear that God can't help me. I once heard a well-renowned life coach tell an audience that fear is a great motivator because if you fear losing your spouse or job, you will treat them much better. I beg to differ. If the only reason I treat my wife well is because I fear losing her, then the only time I will "feel" in love with her is when I fear that our relationship is in trouble. That does not mean I do not understand the position that life coach was trying to portray. As counter-cultural as we are as believers, 1 Corinthians 13:7 tells us that love "bears all things, believes all things, hopes all things, endures all things."

I have had the honor of counseling many singles and couples with flawed ideology, and as I begin to flesh out what ultimately lies beneath all the glitter they present, it comes down to fear. A person can be so consumed with wanting to be loved by someone else that they fool themselves into believing that doing whatever someone wants them to do is love. How mentally sick is that?

What about your job? You might be saying to yourself, "If I fear losing my job, obviously I will work harder." A healthy respect for your job can be a great motivator; however, fear will make you detest the position and the company. And if you put in 20 years of service to only receive a fancy watch with the company logo and a chocolate cake from the nearest supermarket, you may not be afraid to walk out of that job right then in that moment.

The use of fear is different for those who are believers in Christ and those who are not.

"For God has *not* given us a spirit of *fear*, but of power and of love and of a sound mind" (emphasis added) (2 Tim. 1:7).

Did you read that?

If we believe God is in us, we have no space for fear.

I am not saying you will never fear anything, but I am saying that you will conquer all fears through Christ living inside you! You become your thoughts. Counter all negative thoughts you encounter; it is easier than you think.

When I was in college, my long-time roommate and close friend, Brandon, always said, "No worries." I was with Brandon night and day and did not notice when I started to say, "No worries." One night when I was out with my friends, someone at the club accidentally spilled a drink on my white sneakers. I was upset. My mouth was conditioned to respond with "no worries" before my mind could interject with the anger I felt.

"No worries." It became more than a part of my vocabulary; it became an internal mantra that surpassed circumstances and had the easy-flowing response like watching waves roll in an endless ocean.

No worries calmed me.

No worries soothed anxiousness.

No worries responded to fear.

I would like to think that Ivan Pavlov, a Russian physiologist, would have been salivating at my high level of self-conditioning. The person who spilled a drink on my shoe proceeded to clean my shoe with a napkin, and I have no doubt that it was because I gave him a humble response instead of responding with anger. I realized that those two words—no worries—were becoming increasingly powerful. Later, I thought how that scenario could have had a violent outcome. My newfound mind even went a bit further. Why would I wear a white pair of Jordans in a nightclub? It made as much sense as wearing sunglasses in the dark. It took wisdom for me to understand it in retrospect, and I asked myself, "How did I get here?" Proverbs tells us the power of the spoken word. "Death and life are in the power of the tongue. And those who love it will eat its fruit" (Prov. 18:21).

Our words greatly influence our present and our future. That is why Jesus spoke of prayer and communication with God so frequently. Jesus said in James 4:2, "Yet you do not have because you do not ask." Are we asking God to deliver us from fear with the power He is able to do so? When we have fears, they should be met with Scripture such as Proverbs 18:21 and 2 Timothy 1:7.

I encourage you to read them,
to write them down,
to recite them,
to meditate on them,
to memorize them.

Are we asking God to deliver us from fear with the power He is able to do so? When we have fears, they should be met with Scripture.

They will be part of your arsenal when fighting intrusive thoughts. As believers, demons that attempt to attack your mind will not withstand the Word of God coming from your lips. It needs to come from your mouth through prayer, through praise, through worship. There is no fear on earth that Jesus did not cover on the cross. There is also no fear you can carry that will make your life better. "Be anxious for nothing, but in everything by prayer and supplication, with thanksgiving, let your requests be made known to God; and the peace of God, which surpasses all understanding, will guard your hearts and minds through Christ Jesus" (Phil. 4:6–7).

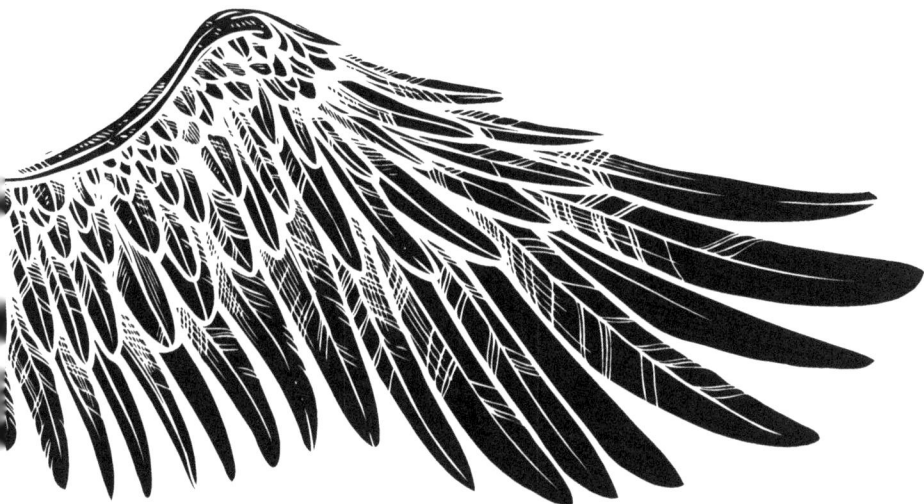

CHAPTER 3

NATURE VS. NURTURE YET AGAIN—IS IT SPIRITUAL WARFARE OR VMAT2?

In 2005, Dean Hamer, an American molecular geneticist, claimed he found the God gene in humans. This was not a new claim, but it was taken more seriously because Hamer was formerly an independent researcher at the National Institutes of Health (NIH) for 35 years where he was chief of the Gene Structure and Regulation Section at the National Cancer Institute. He retired from the NIH in 2011 and wrote a book, *The God Gene: How Faith Is Hardwired into Our Genes*. Hamer argues that a variation in the VMAT2 gene is responsible for our openness to spiritual experiences and predisposition toward spirituality. In the central nervous system, vesicular monoamine transporter 2 (VMAT2) is the only transporter that moves cytoplasmic dopamine into synaptic vesicles for storage and subsequent exocytotic release. He based this on comparing more than 2,000 DNA samples to conclude that belief in God is linked to brain chemicals.

As a rebuttal, Linda A. Silveira (2008) in her article "Experimenting with Spirituality: Analyzing *The God Gene* in a Nonmajors Laboratory Course" expressed that students who conducted the tests Hamer eludes to took a variety of positions. One extreme is becoming adherents of genetic determinism, and at the other extreme is rejecting any role of genetics in human behavior as incompatible with free will.

Silveira argues that in order to believe VMAT2 is responsible for God, you also have to simultaneously believe that genetics are solely responsible for determining a person's characteristics, which would mean the environment plays no role in who you become. Hamer's work has not been published in any scientific journal, although it has been featured in *Time* magazine.

The *New York Times* backed the core of Hamer's findings through science writer Nicholas Wade's notion that 50,000 years ago, religion served as an invisible government that kept those under it committed to a cause, placing the needs of the group ahead of their own. Those gathered to give their lives for their religions would be stronger than those who did not, thus meaning those without the God gene would become extinct.

Fear No Anxiety

Anxiety is common.

It is an unavoidable, inescapable part of life, occasionally.

It is an upcoming exam, that guy at work, potty training, spousal issues, and so on.

An anxiety disorder is literally making a lifetime out of worrying. Anxiety can become a practice that only becomes worse over time.

Generalized anxiety disorders, panic disorders, and various phobia-related disorders are all derived from unchecked fears.

You can go to great lengths to avoid experiencing undesirable emotions or pain, but they will all inevitably fail. They will fail for good reasons. Pain and discomfort are the foundation necessary for incredible growth in this life.

Imagine a seed in the hands of a gardener. The seed is torn from the only home it has ever known and is suddenly riding on the glove of a stranger. The seed thinks to itself, "She seems nice enough." And just when the seed thinks it is safe, it is thrust deep into the ground, buried alive. Maybe the seed screams:

I want to go back to where I came from!

I want to be anywhere but here!

I want to experience anything but this!

To the seed, this is the worst thing that could ever happen. To the gardener, the process cannot be explained to the seed; the gardener just knows.

The seed in all its discomfort starts to feel like it is dying. It complains of the aches and pains and believes the changes to its little body are confirmation of impending doom. It feels the push upward through the dirt as its dramatic exit and last opportunity to smile toward heaven. Suddenly, it notices it has new arms and can see above the soil. It starts growing and can see grass around it and hear the conversations of other busy plants and flowers surrounding it. The gardener comes out, and the sprouting seed sees the gardener smile, pour water over it, tell it to grow, and say how beautiful it is. The seed thinks to itself, I am beautiful, aren't I? I have grown so much! Had I known I would become like this, I would have never made such a fuss with all that worry.

What the seed did not know until that moment is that it was meant to be more than a mere seed. The gardener knew what the seed would become in due time. God knew what you would become before you were ever born. He never got worried, anxious, or impatient. He knew what you would not understand, so He planted you on the earth to grow! All your questions and all your concerns will not stop or alter what you are here to become unless you allow your worries to consume you to the point of refusing to be planted. Yes, it is uncomfortable. Yes, it is painful at times. Yes, it is not what you planned. Yet it is everything you had no idea would get you where God wanted you to be—a life with a more fulfilling purpose than you ever imagined for yourself. Trust that God's plan for your life, even through discomfort, is greater and has more purpose than your own plan.

Your plan has too much you in it.
His plan has just enough you, him, her,
them, us, and we for the Kingdom!

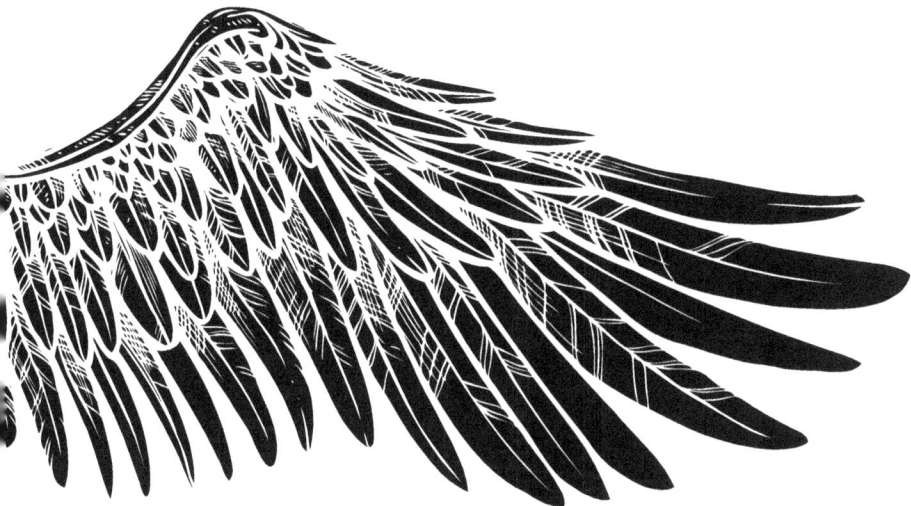

CHAPTER 4

JESUS DIAGNOSED

And he took with Him Peter and the two sons of Zebedee, and He began to be sorrowful and deeply distressed.

—Matt. 26:37

This portion of the book, this very section of the book, has provided me with quite a few restless nights. This section on Jesus Christ and what the mental health field feels about Jesus—three years of Jesus's life, the Gospel ages of 30 to 33 when He preached the Word of God, died for all people's sins, and rose again on the third day—is the most controversial topic in the world.

---

*No matter which psychiatrist I spoke with,
the mention of Jesus Christ brought a kaleidoscope
of responses.*

Maybe it was the responses—scoffing, laughing, looking at me puzzled. Some immediately went into a thinking-man's pose with the hand beneath the chin in deep thought. I want to share with you the best two answers, one from a well-renowned psychiatrist in the field who made a name for himself by creating his own theologies, and the other from a psychiatrist who is well-known as a patient's psychiatrist. He spends a lot of time with his patients and is reluctant to add medications to a patient's chart without discussing the side effects with patients and staff.

The first response I chose was due to how big this psychiatrist is across the mental health community. He has been on the cover of magazines, a guest on TED Talks, and a *New York Times* best-selling author. He has flown around the world to speak to large audiences and all that jazz. I called his office numerous times as well as showed up in person in order to lock down a lunch interview. I sweetened the deal by stating, "One lunch on me, only a handful of questions, you can pick any restaurant near your office (Newport Beach, California), and I will be done with my questions by the time the food is at the table."

After months of pleading, he agreed, and just like that, there I sat at Tommy Bahama, hoping he showed up since he was 15 minutes late and had stated he only had 30 minutes to spare. I had already ordered my second glass of water on the rocks, shaken, not stirred, nervously looking at the menu to find the most affordable options when out the window I spotted his black, matte-finished Porsche Panamera GTS. There was this air about him; you felt like he was important and almost vetted your words before speaking.

Dr. Gold

I stood up and held out my hand, and it appeared he reluctantly shook it. I passed it off as being a COVID-19 precaution and not a hierarchy concern. He had on an expensive blue suit, tapioca Aldo shoes, a striped tie, and a fancy gold handkerchief. I recall this, not because it was so impressive, but because it was underwhelming, predictable, like googling "psychiatrist," as if he were wearing a psychiatrist skin suit or something.

I would not have dared say anything about that, though, because I needed this highly esteemed opinion, and of course, I had no clue what he would say. He could be for, against, or surprise me all the same. The topic intrigued him, yet the first thing he did was demand that I leave his practice and real name out of his response. I smiled because I knew that not only were the words coming out of his mouth about to be biased but that he would only stand behind them so far so he would not put his illustrious career at any risk.

So Dr. "Gold" started out by saying he was well versed in the stories of Christ and the Gospels because he grew up with a distant relative who was very religious in the Catholic faith but could not become a priest because of his expressed homosexuality. I thought that was quite the beginning. He ordered a scotch on the rocks, and I splurged on a root beer in a tall glass. He went on. "Let's take out titles because titles always make things more than they need to be." (I would love to point out that Dr. Gold has a personalized license plate, but I fear he would be found out quickly.) Here is what Dr. Gold said (from a transcript of the recording):

> *Let's just look at it like this. He is 100 percent human.*
> *We have a guy who was born and raised in Bethlehem*
> *by Mary and Joseph. Joseph was a humble carpenter;*
> *Mary was religious. We are not going to speculate on*
> *the absurdity of Mary being a virgin impregnated by*

a "spirit" or how he was a carpenter by trade who all of a sudden has endless supernatural powers, is the son of God, heals people, brings people back from the dead, performs deliverances or exorcisms or whatever you want to call them. He still has time to turn water to wine at weddings, knows more about God than the Pharisees at age nine, teaching Pharisees in a temple [scoffs] when it is their profession. He hears the voice of God speak to him, he sees angels, knows things before his time, and honestly, if you were to pick one event, choose where he is begging God not to have to go to a cross he does not want to go to and ends up bleeding through his pores in anxiety.

He chuckled while throwing his arms in the air and continued. "I mean, you have to admit, there is so much to go on here!"

I will admit that in that albeit brief rant, I was surprised at how much he researched, even if taken out of context. He had more familiarity about Christ than most psychiatrists I had met. It beckoned me to wonder about his fascination about religion. I wanted to interject and provide my opinion, but two things stopped me. First, this was not about me; it was about the book, and I wanted him to feel free to have his own opinion. Second, I literally was not afforded the opportunity to provide my opinion since he had so much to say without taking a breath.

I wanted more, so I did what I thought a smart journalist would do and told him, "Wow! That is fascinating. I have not met a psychiatrist who has that much knowledge about the Bible. Where did you learn so much?"

He responded, "Not how; why did I learn so much? I wanted to know why people dedicate themselves to fantasies or hang on to a better life than the one they can create themselves. Why wait for an invisible being to approve of you moving forward with your life?"

Just then the waiter popped up, and Dr. Gold ordered seared scallops, and I ordered ahi tuna. He ordered another scotch and then went on about Jesus as if he had been thinking the whole time.

If it were just the one sweat-to-bleeding incident, you could write it off as anxiety, write him a prescription of Buspar or Clonidine and be done with it, but there are the hallucinations of seeing the unseen, the delusions of grandeur, the Son of God, are not we all? I mean, Jesus Christ [realizes what he just said and laughs]! It is almost too easy to say he would be the textbook delusional disorder case. How is he any different than any other cult leader like [David] Koresh or [Jim] Jones?

It felt like the lights just went out in Tommy Bahama. Not only did Dr. Gold diagnose Jesus Christ, he lumped him in the same cult category with David Koresh and Jim Jones. David Koresh and Jim Jones? As a reader, imagine you have been told that this guy Dr. Gold is the golden standard in the psychiatric field. To hear him say this is like a Catholic being flipped off by the Pope. This is the same man who prescribes you psych meds, the same man you trust to diagnose you because he graduated in 1977 from a then-prestigious school. If you think you have a right to be offended by psychiatrists who diagnose you within less than five minutes of meeting you, imagine a psychiatrist who has the power to diagnose you through the five-minute interactions of his intern staff. I know, I was bitter.

At that point, I still could not believe David Koresh and Jim Jones came out of Dr. Gold's mouth. They were cult leaders with no similarities to Jesus Christ. They sacrificed their own followers, while Jesus Christ (God in flesh) sacrificed His own life. Neither Koresh nor Jones rose again on the third day. Those are just the obvious differences. Even if Dr. Gold was not a believer in Jesus Christ or God, it flowed easily off his tongue as if there was no hesitation or doubt in his mind that nearly everyone felt like he did. It was a hard hit to take, yet Christianity equaling lunacy is a spreading theme in our modern world.

From that point on, I was in and out of hearing Dr. Gold's words as he rambled on about how blind faith is archaic and baseless, and religion throughout history has "herded people and provided hope for those afraid of taking responsibility for their own actions or unwilling to take life by the horns." Dr. Gold stated that religiosity provides hope that the next life will be better—heaven, reincarnation, 40 virgins—all the same garbage wrapped in different shrapnel. The hits just kept coming. I am used to this perspective in the mental health field. As far back as sitting in undergrad courses in psychology at Long Beach State, I witnessed the same treatment of faith. In graduate courses during my third master's degree at Grand Canyon University, I recall a group discussion where a topic on abortion got so heated that the pro-choice students threatened to communicate to the dean in regard to pro-life positions. Mind you, Grand Canyon University is a faith-based university. Dr. Gold was still in the background as I was diving through the archives of personal experiences in my mind.

I did not find my distance learning with Dr. Gold when it came to being rude. He needed no audience, just an opportunity to hear his fantastic thoughts out loud. I just happened to look down at my watch and realized we had hit the two-hour mark on Dr. Gold's strict 30 minutes of availability. I had what I was seeking, so I ended the conversation by exclaiming, "I am so sorry, Dr. Gold. I have completely lost track of time and by no means wanted to disrespect the thirty minutes you promised me." Apparently, he liked me since he shook my hand like we were old hood-and-cloak brothers, reminded me not to use his name in my book, and then told me, "If the book gets done, go ahead and send me a copy. It would be cool. Let's do this again to celebrate." I will be personally signing a copy and handing it to him. I'm not a monster. I pray for his salvation, a road-to-Damascus experience where his Panamera talks to him.

I keep a digital copy in my phone of the *Diagnostic and Statistical Manual* (*DSM-5*), the Kelley Blue Book of mental illness. You never know when you will need to verify someone's claim or cross-diagnose, check symptoms, and so on. The *DSM* previously was a much more respected measure of mental issues until pharmaceutical companies helped *DSM* with its decision-making process when it comes to criteria. It was great for big pharmaceuticals, not so great for patients and mental health workers scrambling to make circles fit in holes meant for triangles. Albeit it is still useful for cross-checking.

Delusional disorder, previously called paranoid disorder—the stand-out of this disorder is that delusional disorder is classified as a psychosis where a person cannot tell what is real from what is imagined. It is impossible to convince this person that what they believe is not true. For this criterion, the experiences people have had are non-bizarre delusions miscommunicated as reality. The experiences are either not true at all or highly exaggerated. Yet biblically speaking, there are many stories corroborating Jesus Christ and His miracles outside of Himself.

The story that immediately stands out to me is the man born blind whom Jesus healed in John 9. Jesus Christ heals this man who had been blind from birth. If Jesus were suffering from delusional disorder, He would have been the only one to believe He healed the man, considering it would fit the self-serving grandiose label. Jesus Christ heals the man, and then the man tells people about what happened to him, and the miracle reaches the doors of the Pharisees who have a lot to lose if Jesus is the Lamb of God and delivers people from their blind allegiance to the Pharisees. They want to dispel the healing of the blind man by bringing the man in and asking him a series of questions regarding Christ in hopes of discrediting the miracle.

If it were a delusional disorder, then why were there so many people who not only witnessed it but told the Pharisees as well? If others witnessed the miracles, then how are they delusional? How are they grandiose?

I had to look up the criteria for delusional disorder (grandiose) in detail. That way, you as a reader can make your own judgment on Jesus Christ. Here are the symptoms Jesus Christ displayed according to the *DSM-5*:

1. Delusional disorder (grandiose type). There are a few types, but the diagnosis for Jesus Christ would be grandiose, which means a person with this type of delusional disorder has an overinflated sense of worth, power, knowledge, or identity. The person might believe he or she has a great talent or has made an important discovery.
2. Visual and auditory hallucinations
3. Referential thought process

If you were to cross-reference Scriptures that could be used to back this possibility, paranoid-type (PS subtype) thought content could be argued by the following verses:

Matthew 10:34–39, 16:21–23, 24:4–27; Mark 13:5–6; Luke 10:19; John 3:18, 14:6–11; Matthew 3:16–17, 4:3–11.

Auditory and visual hallucinations could be argued by the following verses: Luke 10:18; John 6:46, 8:26, 8:38–40, 12:28–29.

Referential thought processes could be argued by the following verse: Luke 18:31.

I shudder to think what would have happened if, indeed, Jesus had been seen praying until he sweat droplets of blood that fateful night in Gethsemane. What if it were played out today? Would Jesus be met by a psychiatric team off a 9-1-1 call by someone named Karen? What if our Lord and Savior never made it to the cross because the adjustments to his medications were too much? Some lab coat walks in and immediately assumes Jesus has a serotonin issue or some other neurotransmitter concern and pumps Him full of risperidone (Risperdal), clozapine (Clozaril), quetiapine (Seroquel), ziprasidone (Geodon), or olanzapine (Zyprexa). Would Jesus be strapped to a metal bed, shipped to Mission Hospital's mental health unit, and drugged up? I am forever grateful that we did not have to experience that since, of course, there would have been no *us*.

When you are looking at depression, Jesus showed us as God in the flesh what depression and anxiety look like in the Gospels alone. He fought depression by having a support team (Matt. 26:37), He was open and honest about what He was feeling (Matt. 26:38), He prayed and asked for His support team to pray for Him (Matt. 26:38), He prayed to the Father (Matt. 26:39), and He left it all ultimately in God's hands (Matt. 26:39).

Dr. Littman

Dr. Littman is the second psychiatrist whose opinion stood out to me. He is a psychiatrist, like Dr. Gold, who claimed to be a Christian and know the Bible. He works in a psychiatric hospital in Newport Beach, California. Dr. Littman is in his late 40s and Caucasian. He has dark hair and deep brown eyes. He appears busy, even when he is standing still doing nothing at all, yet he also has an internal drive that only genius people have. He does not want the responsibility of being the only one with answers in the room, yet he knows if he doesn't provide the answer, no one else will. Dr. Gold was the type of doctor who would crush your soul with his piety if you said the wrong thing in an interdisciplinary team meeting, proving how intelligent he was.

Dr. Littman, however, is the type of doctor who would go to great lengths to prove how you came to your answer and how much sense it makes, yet urge you to go deeper and find the root in a way that makes you feel smarter.

Dr. Littman did not hesitate to profess that he is a Christian. He wanted me to know that in case I could not use his opinion since it was biased. This caught my attention, especially in a day and age where faith and career seem to be dividing at an all-time high. Dr. Littman had the upper hand of hearing my previous interview with Dr. Gold and asked me to read the transcript. After a long pause, he started laughing aloud. I could not help laughing as well, but then he asked me what I thought while Jesus was being diagnosed. I stopped laughing. I said it was scary. I told him it reminded me of a book I once read, *Foxe's Book of Martyrs*, and I thought of the incredible extents people have gone to in order to try to eradicate God, Jesus, religion, and faith.

A doctor who asked my opinion before giving me his—what a great start! I told him it was tough to hear Dr. Gold speak so little of Jesus Christ as if He had no importance at all. Dr. Littman provided me with nonverbal agreement with head nods, and then he replied, "Antonio, as a psychiatrist, you are looking at symptoms, not the person. You and I would see that scene differently because of the narrative we have accepted. We have accepted Jesus Christ as being the Son of God and it being necessary for Him to carry out His death on the cross knowing that He was doing so for our sins, and resurrecting on the third day. In other words, we take Jesus personal, so we take what is said about Him personal as well."

There it was, the Willy Wonka golden ticket placed in my hand. Narrative. This narrative theme would play out. Jesus knew who He was, what He was on earth for, and what He had to do. He knew He had to be sacrificed in order to save those who answered the knock at their hearts for an all-expenses-paid trip to heaven for eternity. He accepted taking on the ultimate mental stressors available to mankind on our behalf. He was "labeled," so when you are labeled or diagnosed, remember that He told us we would be persecuted for His name's sake.

Blessed are those who are persecuted for righteousness' sake, for theirs is the kingdom of heaven. Blessed are you when they revile and persecute you, and say all kinds of evil against you falsely for My sake. Rejoice and be exceedingly glad, for great is your reward in heaven, for so they persecuted the prophets who were before you.

—Matt. 5:10–12

He had to be sacrificed in order to save those who answered the knock at their hearts for an all-expenses-paid trip to heaven for eternity.

Why does that fit in the face of what you are facing? "For the message of the cross is foolishness to those who are perishing, but to us who are being saved it is the power of God" (1 Cor. 1:18).

Even your mental health is in God's hands. He knows what you are going through. He is for you and not against you!

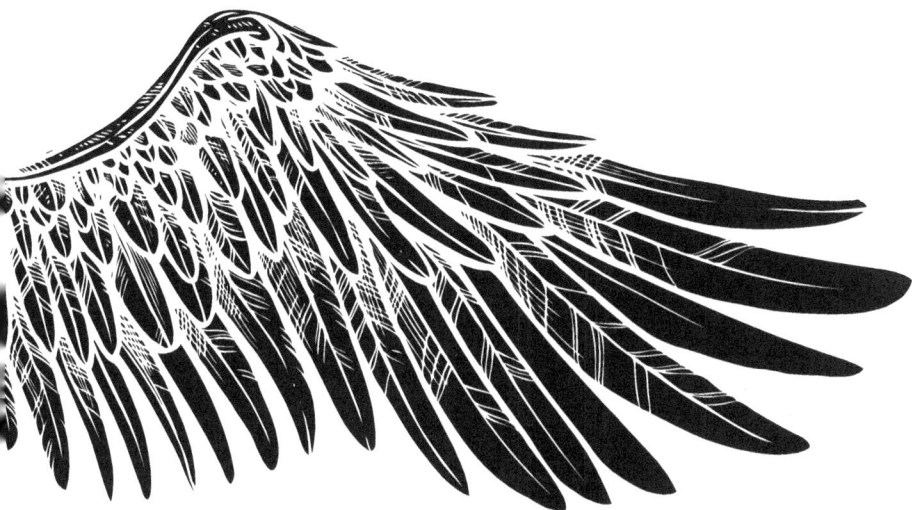

CHAPTER 5

INTRODUCING THE HYPER-RELIGIOUS LABEL

I formerly worked as a patients' rights advocate (PRA) in Orange County. I worked for 13 mental health units (hospitals) and the Orange County jail. I was not in that position long, but the amount of corruption was so toxic from so many angles that when I approached the CEO regarding how politically horrid the inner workings of the organizations were, I was let go immediately. I was not surprised. I just could not be silent any longer about the injustices that were taking place. My move was met by applause and respect from my great mentors in the field.

One of my former positions was to argue if a mental health unit had the right to keep a client on a hold against their will through medical necessity in a certified hearing. I represented the patient, and a social worker or doctor would argue for the unit. In this case, a patient is placed on a 72-hour hold (5150) first. If they are not released from that hold, they are provided a certified hearing, which allows the patient the opportunity to let the hearing officer know what got them on a hold and what steps they are taking so it will not occur again. I am not going to tell you that everyone I encountered should not have been on a hold. On the contrary, many people I attempted to represent were looking for "three hots and a cot" (three meals and lodging) or were so caught up in guilt and depression that they wanted to remain in a locked psychiatric unit.

Yet there were cases that kept me up at night as the census got low in mental health units. Calls were made, and they were filled to the brim within hours. Psychiatrists and social workers alike would cringe when they heard that officers and patients' rights advocates had arrived because it meant any hold that did not meet a medical necessity would be argued. On many occasions, it appeared as though hearing officers and patients' rights advocates were the cavalry for mental health patients. Many days, the hearing officer and I would start at 8:30 a.m. and not finish four or more unit facilities until 8:00 p.m. or later. It was never pretty, but it was always worth it.

Within my first three months of working as a PRA, I was able to read a hold written by a psychiatrist and guess which therapist wrote the hold by the diagnosis. Oddly enough, psychiatrists have the tendency to write holds based on their specialties and expertise. Hence, if a psychiatrist has a specialty in schizophrenia, suddenly there is a surge in schizophrenia or dementia diagnoses. Knowing a psychiatrist by their narratives might sound like quite a feat across 13 facilities, but Orange County's mental health community is smaller than you would imagine. It was not uncommon for me to see the same psychiatrists' names pop up on the spines of patients' binders across three facilities in one day.

The biggest complaint I received was that patients reported never having met a psychiatrist and being given a hold in under 5–10 minutes with a diagnosis and medication. The psychiatrist never got the narrative of the client or other substantial information, which would have been a better determinant of the patient's behavior. It is painfully obvious that it would be hard to get to three hospitals and write medications for patients if you were not quick and robotic in your technique. Doesn't that feel wrong?

Do you know how a 5150 that leads to a 5250 (14-day additional hold) affects a person's life? It follows them when they attempt to continue school, obtain certain positions in their career (especially government positions), or have an apartment of their own when mental illness can be part of a background check. I will share the patient's story that led to the first conversation sparking my interest in writing this book. I had a client admitted to an eminent mental health hospital because she said in an emergency room, "I am so upset I could just kill myself right now!" She later stated that she said it out of frustration and did not have the means to desperately cry out to anyone who would listen. Yet at her hearing, because she refused to take the psychiatrist's suggested medications and appeared labile and depressed, she received a 5250, 14 days more after already spending 72 hours on an initial 5150 hold.

I asked the social worker representing the busily absent psychiatrist if, in the patient's shoes, she also might feel labile and depressed. That was the only thing holding the client, according to the psychiatrist. I asked the social worker representing the hospital if she thought being labile and depressed was strong enough for a 14-day hold, knowing that is not enough to meet medical necessity, especially when the client has family present who are willing to take her home with them. The client was Asian, and saying you want to die or harm yourself in many cultures is not a profession of suicidal ideology as is widely accepted in Western civilization. I had seen nothing in the staff that accounted for cultural competency or awareness.

If that was not enough, I had an ace in my pocket since the client was three months pregnant. She said it had fallen on deaf ears in the emergency room after her car accident and also in the mental health unit. So I asked the attending social worker if there were any tests or measures taken to account for the possibility of postpartum depression and why being pregnant was not a suitable reason for the client to not only refuse medications but also a reason for the client to be currently labile and depressed. Both are symptoms of postpartum depression. The social worker was confused since it was most likely the first time she had heard that the patient was pregnant. She admitted there was nothing in the records of a pregnancy test being administered to my client.

I would not have approached the case so violently, but I was upset at the entire system at that moment. The social worker left to get another social worker who called the lead psychiatrist. Nonetheless, I won that case, and the patient was released immediately. The mother of this patient, Dr. Pham, found me in the lobby and pursued an intriguing conversation.

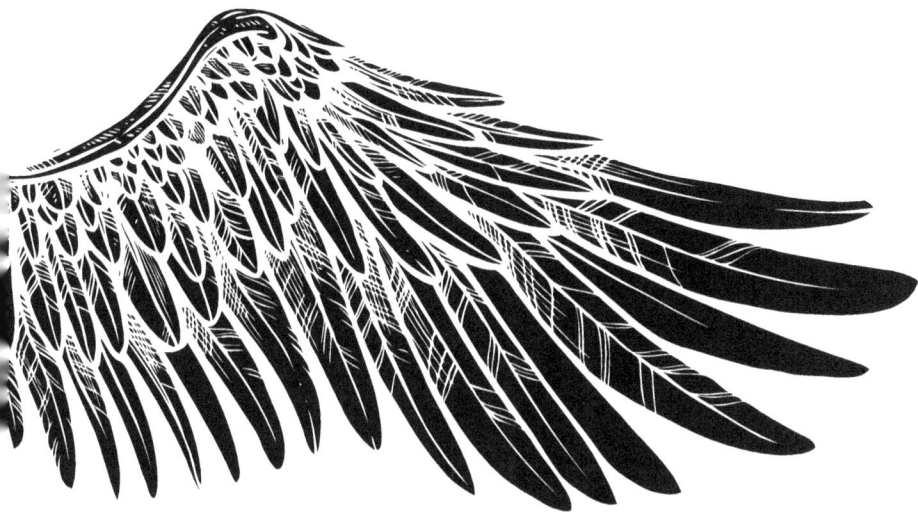

CHAPTER 6

THE STORY OF DR. PHAM

Dr. Pham was born in a small farm village in North Vietnam with generations of rice farmers on both sides. She said that all she knew was small life, chickens, fish, water buffalo, and helping in the fields. They were not rich or poor, but both parents worked hard. In 1954, when she was five years old, Vietnam split into the north and the south. Fearing being killed by communists, her family boarded an American ship and went from North Vietnam to South Vietnam.

I asked Dr. Pham how they ended up becoming Catholics, and she stated that her mother and father cut trees and sold wood in South Vietnam to build schools, and one day a missionary visited her parents. She said the missionary talked to the entire village, and they converted to Catholicism.

By age 18, Dr, Pham took a vow to become a nun. The Dominican Order was close to the American GI base, and the American chaplain came there to teach English to the students. He brought soldiers who taught songs during mass in both languages. They brought snacks for the children and prepared vestments for the services. After a year, Dr. Pham's family had learned conversational English. They learned how to read and write, and they increased their vocabulary and improved their grammar. When they were leaving Vietnam, they were asked if they needed anything. Dr. Pham raised her hand and asked if they would be willing to provide scholarships for the nuns to learn English in America, and the American chaplain brought four of the nuns with him, including Dr. Pham, and paid for their tickets. Dr. Pham landed in Michigan on August 28, 1968. She received a bachelor's degree and moved to Pennsylvania where she received a master's degree in 1973 and started training at Boston's Westborough State Hospital for a clinical pastoral degree. Most of the people who completed the degree became hospital administrators and chaplains.

In 1976, Dr. Pham married a Buddhist from Vietnam. Although she was marrying a man who was not Catholic, they could get married in a Catholic church. To this day she states that her husband still considers himself a Buddhist although he attends church with her every Sunday. In 1979, they had their first child, Dominique, named after the Dominicans who rescued her from her village. Then they had Michelle in 1982, and Andrea was born in 1983.

In 1979, Dr. Pham received her doctoral degree from the University of Houston. She laughs when she remembers that at the time it was only $300 per semester. Dr. Pham felt she had a calling to lead people onto their paths, and with all the faith within her, she applied in 1985 to a counseling position at a prestigious college in Southern California. Within months, her family left Houston and moved to Southern California. When people asked why, she said, "The weather is close to heaven!" I included the amount of information I did of Dr. Pham's life because her experience warrants attention when she speaks. Even a few words from Dr. Pham are laced in wisdom. She told me the following regarding mental health:

> *I look at mental health or illness as any type of illness. Cancer attacks certain types of the body; mental illnesses attack a part of the body, the mind. Mental illness can be helped by faith. I tell my own daughter who struggles with mental illness to pray. She tells her daughter to have faith and pray to God. With faith you will always survive. If you lose faith, you lose your life. There are too many stigmas attached with mental illness. They keep those who are needing help from receiving it. If someone tells the company, I found out I have cancer, everyone rallies to help that person and give them hope. When someone says I have schizophrenia or some other mental illness, people flee as if the person suffering caused it or that it can spread through touch or conversation. I understand faith in not having medication, but you cannot win a lottery without buying a ticket. What if God wants to heal you through the medication? If you don't accept it, you could be missing out on the lottery of your mental health.*

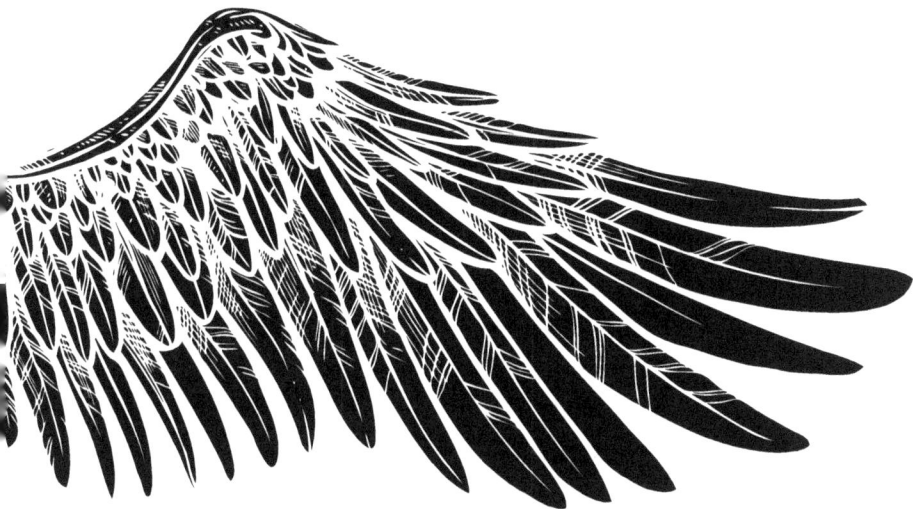

CHAPTER 7

MUST BE THE SEASON OF THE WITCH

Case Studies

I had a stretch of clients who were claiming to have auditory or visual hallucinations of being chased by witches. If you work in mental health, that is not profound or unique; many patients believe that. You will come across a lot of patients claiming they are FBI agents, CIA agents, God, the devil, angels, demons, and more. I have yet to run across a patient who claimed they were someone of little to no importance. One case followed me through three hospitals and caused me some sleepless nights. The woman, Hala, was from Jordan.

Hala claimed she had two teenage sons who were kidnapped and murdered because she refused to leave the Christian faith when she was in a Muslim community. She said once it was confirmed they were dead, she had no reason to remain in Jordan tortured by their memories, so she did what she had to do and came to America. Hala was the type of patient you hoped you did not run into. She wandered the hallways of the mental health ward, disheveled, appearing in physical pain, weeping aloud, asking anyone who cared to listen to her, "Please, can you help me?"

My cape was on fire; I had to listen to her story. The first question I asked her was how she got to the mental health hospital. She stated that she was taken in because she ran into traffic, and the police said she was a danger to herself and others. Hala then went on to tell me that since she left Jordan, even on the plane, she started feeling a dark presence around her. She said she felt it but did not see anything until one night in her bedroom. High on the ceiling in a corner was a dark entity that moved without a shadow.

Hala said it was not like the darkness that is nighttime; it was evil and just stared at her. She said she first saw the witch behind her in a mirror and did not say anything because she knew people would think she was crazy. The witch remained in her home, popping up periodically, saying nothing, and just staring at Hala. The day in question, Hala had just gotten off a bus in Garden Grove and was heading to her apartment when she heard fast-moving feet behind her from a distance. She turned to see the witch chasing her and screaming that she must die.

Hala said she was scared for her life because the witch had only been in the house, and now it was outside chasing her and speaking words. Hala said she was not trying to commit suicide; she was trying to get help when she ran across the busy street. She said no one believed her, and they would not let her out of the hospital. I saw that the psychiatrist had placed her on Haldol as one of her medications. She claimed she was seeing the witch even as we spoke. I started praying for Hala. I wanted her to know that I believed something had happened to her. Hala ended up in three psychiatric hospitals and was placed on holds at all three as she tried to get away from the witch.

Within a month's time, she aged rapidly. She progressed from a 72-hour hold to a 14-day hold to a 30-day hold to a long-term facility, and the last time I saw Hala, she was at peace. Her skin was glowing, and she smiled when she saw me. She was not wandering the hallways or weeping. She simply told me that she was okay and was not seeing the witch anymore.

The staff reported that since being in the long-term facility, Hala had refused medications, and since she exhibited no symptoms, no agitations, and no aggressive behavior, they were not going to push her for more medications and were going to discharge her. My flesh was confused. From a medical standpoint, it seemed hopeless, yet in my faith I saw God working, not in the first prayer, not in the second, but with continuous prayer. Not only does it grow the faith of the person praying, but it also grows the warrior inside the believer.

How do we deal with our mental health? We use substances to numb the pain and people to numb the pain, which only makes hurting people hurt people. We have turned "I am blessed," as a false response, masking what we are enduring.

A coping mechanism used incorrectly
becomes nothing more than a Band-Aid
on a fatal wound.

So many things can be placed to temporarily fill a void. If you continue to ignore the root of the problem, you will continue to live an empty life that no amount of coping mechanisms can fill. It makes sense when you think about it. You are counting on something that is empty to fill an emptiness. Can you imagine coming across someone in the desert who is dying of thirst and offering them an empty water bottle? It would not make any sense. If you were the one who was hoping for water, you would be angry or at least confused.

Winning Over Jonah and Tio
Jonah

Short intro here. After a forever vow was cut awfully short at a burning altar, I made a larger vow to never be married again and made a list so big of what I wanted that I knew the woman would not exist, and if she did, she was not looking for me. God thought I was funny and introduced me to my wife through a tacky online dating site I would have bet He was not paying any attention to. After months of online conversation, we had our first date, walking along the beach in Long Beach, California, across the street from my future studio apartment on Ocean Beach. We had hot cocoa I made myself and walked and talked all night about everything from God and spiritual warfare to '80s pop culture. I knew when I got home that night that I was in trouble. I already liked Adriana too much, but that entire story is for the next book. I mention it because we ended up getting married and moving in with her family since I could not stay away from her and my incredible son, Kareem, through God's union. I moved in with my wife's family in Santa Ana. What I thought would be a year and a half tops ended up being four years before we moved out on our own. I always wanted a big family, so it really was a great experience for me to live with 10 people in a five-bedroom house, even if only half of them spoke English.

When we moved in, I prayed with my wife to lead every member of the household to Christ who did not know Him. Jonah was dating my wife's cousin Lina, and I knew that both Jonah and Lina's father would be a challenge to talk to about the gospel.

I would describe Jonah like Thor. He was about 6'4" with blond hair, blue sharp eyes, and 250 pounds of troubled past. Jonah was quiet and reserved and appeared to have no interest whatsoever. I recall holding Bible studies at the table in hopes that Jonah would join us. He did so a few times, and I even played some short stories on YouTube that talked about the history of Jesus Christ.

God works in mysterious ways. A mysterious way in our home was Tio, Lina's father, the alpha male of Adriana's family who became severely ill after his blood was poisoned during dialysis. My mother-in-law called and asked me to pray for Tio Beto who was in the hospital. I had just met him a few weeks earlier, yet I had heard a lot about him and respected him greatly. I was nervous, but I knew I did not need to know him to pray for his situation. As we walked into the hospital room, I could feel the great amount of respect the family had for Tio Beto. The doctor did not see Beto lasting long since his oxygen had reached a point of no return, according to his paperwork.

Tio Beto's family from all sides was coming to see him. They were from Mexico and Northern California, a bunch of twenty-somethings who rarely attended family functions but sat in silence at his bedside. They believed he was on death's doorstep. I was still new to the family, and I recall Adriana's mother asking me to please pray for Beto. I anointed his hands and his head, and I prayed for him daily. Two weeks later, Tito Beto walked out of the hospital like nothing had happened.

My wife and I were blessed to have the opportunity to take him out to eat, and I shared the gospel with him. He had been listening to Bible studies and wanted Jesus in his life. He said one of the things that stood out to him was that he did not ask God why it happened; he just adjusted. That day in a restaurant he prayed, and a seed was planted. His daughter Lina would follow her father soon after one random day, kneeling beside me and my wife, calling out to God. Adriana's aunt Angelica would follow and attend the Spanish church connected to our church. Jonah was the only one left of the original core I had prayed for.

As time rolled by, I tried movies, clips, Scripture, scenarios, and more. Nothing worked to move Jonah. He talked about his history in prison. He talked about missing his daughter, a toddler living with her mother. He talked about his past with alcohol and drugs, but he would not talk about accepting Christ. He went so far as to tell me, "Look, I just don't want to talk about that stuff, so drop it." Oddly, his stubborn nature only made me want to see God in his life that much more. Abruptly, Jonah and Lina decided to get their own apartment, and I told Jonah they needed to get married and get counseling to better secure that bond. They left anyway. It lasted about six months, and then they split up. I knew something was up because Lina showed up for the holidays that year solo, and the story of Jonah being "on call all the time" did not add up for a guy who felt like he only had us as family. My heart resonated for Jonah because he once told me he never had a family and that if he lost Lina, he would lose not just her but an entire family he had come to love and trust.

Let's fast-forward. Lina and Jonah broke up, Jonah had a few friends pass away, and he was renting a room on the other side of town. He slipped into a deep depression, and he figured that Xanax and alcohol were great coping mechanisms. Then he called me. I was surprised that he called me at all. We talked for a while, and I did not mention Christ. I just listened to him talk. He was slurring so much and was so incoherent that I could not make much of what he was saying. That continued for about two days before I could clearly hear him talk one night.

It was that night that I told Jonah he was drowning, and he admitted he was having suicidal thoughts. He would not let me come to him and would not allow me to call a psychiatric evaluation team to assess him. I had a brother at church who had been through many similar issues and struggles, and Jonah called and talked to him. I then asked Jonah over the phone if he was ready to try Christ, especially since doing things his own way had not worked well in the last 27 years. He mumbled something in frustration and hung up the phone.

On the following morning, my phone got a ding, and it was Jonah. He asked me to talk with him about Christ and that he was sorry he had hung up on me the previous night. I forgave him and said, "Let's hang out." Jonah did not contact me for two days, but he had given me cues that I needed to pray for his battle. Jonah was now crossing from mental illness to spiritual warfare. I was heading to Jonah's when he asked me to get him some ice cream. I bought him two ice creams from 7-Eleven.

As I was arriving, I got another ding from Jonah who was upset that I was taking so long and to forget about it. I smiled. The spiritual battle was afoot. I pulled up to his place, and Jonah stumbled toward my car. At the time, Jonah was 6'4" and around 300 pounds. When he got in the car, he was profusely sweating and appeared in pain and under the influence. I drove him around the corner to a parking lot and heard about all the pain and anger inside of him.

I listened patiently to Jonah's words, but I could not hear him above the Holy Spirit speaking. I listened intently.

I then told Jonah that I only knew of one thing that could fix it all, and that was surrendering to Jesus Christ.

Jonah then went into how many times he had tried but just could not give his life to Christ. I put my arm on Jonah's shoulder as he started crying about how he did not want to hurt anymore and was done fighting. Surrender.

I said to him, "If you want to pray this prayer with me, nothing you will go through on this earth will be without a purpose greater than yourself, and you will have peace in the middle of the storm." I said these words and still get goose bumps today as I remember the tears rolling down both of our faces that day. Jonah prayed, "Jesus, I believe that you died for my sins and rose again on the third day. I repent of all my sins and want you to come into my life, lead my life, direct my path, and use me for your glory. I am yours. Amen."

I had another prayer in my head, but the emotions were so thick and the Holy Spirit so present that lengthy prayers were unnecessary. Jonah needed to feel God's love that day—pure, unfiltered, unconditional love. I cautioned Jonah that life as a Christian does not mean everything is immediately peaches and cream but that finally, with his salvation, he provided Christ the opportunity to fight on his behalf.

A week passed before Jonah contacted me. He told me he had been on the floor of his rented room for four days, unable to get up. My wife was on a trip to Big Bear with friends, and I had no one to watch our three-year-old daughter, so I took her with me and kept her by my side. I rushed to Jonah's place and found him laid out on the floor wearing only boxers. He could talk, but even the slightest movement made him scream in excruciating pain.

His room was very smelly, and I found that he had urinated in small water bottles because he could not get up. There were also aluminum foil with burn marks, a small pipe in the window, and bottles of various alcohol everywhere. I called an ambulance to pick him up, cleaned up his room, and put everything in bags. It was time for Jonah to get in the whale and live out his true purpose.

Jonah had a childhood friend who gave her life to God at a young age. She stated that she had been through all the drug and alcohol wars with her father and one of her brothers and that she was ready for Jonah to move from California to Chicago where she lived and put him through rehabilitation. The next day, my daughter and I took Jonah to the train station in Fullerton. Jonah thanked me, I prayed with him, and then I sent him off with love and some money for food. Jonah's friend called me and texted me about how exciting it would be to see the new Jonah in a few months. I am writing this the same day he boarded the train. I trust God above all circumstances and know that Jonah's story is a testimony. Jonah would be one of the most personal stories I have dealt with to date.

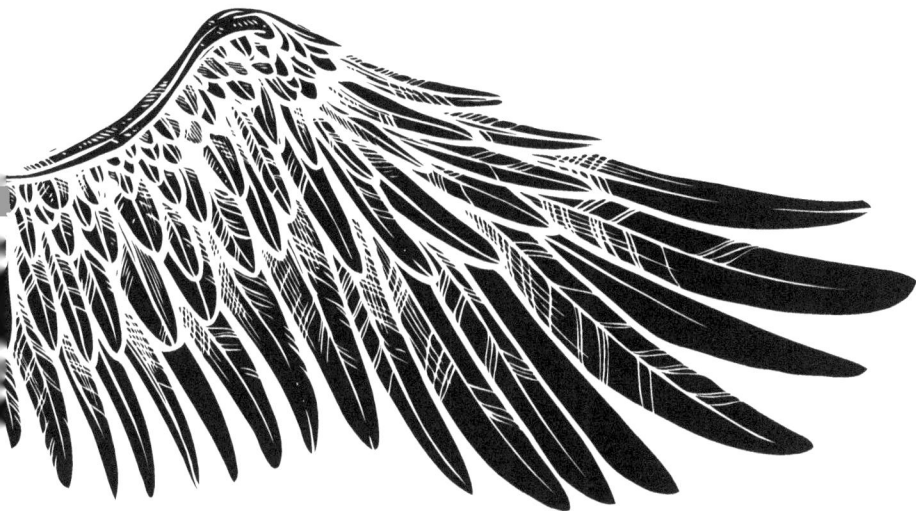

CHAPTER 8

"THE BLACK MESSIAH"

Rock is another big boy, about 6'4" and 300 pounds, Black, and born and raised in Southern California but now living with his wife and three children in Georgia. Rock is street intelligent through self-research and severe paranoia. This internal struggle creates massive amounts of deep mistrust in Rock's mind. He was about 30 when I met him, and I was highly anticipating meeting another "brother" in the family. Our first conversation did not go as planned on the phone when we talked about possible things we had in common. No, I don't smoke marijuana. No, I don't shoot pool. No, I don't play dominoes. No, I don't play cards. Rock seemed disappointed that I was not like him, and I was disappointed that those were his defining qualities of friendship. He went on to presume what type of person I was, and of course,

I could not understand why he would not just ask me since we were talking on the phone.

At that point, I was not sure if we were going to like each other at all. Still, I like to keep a positive mind about things, so when Rock and the family came to visit, I was open and positive. Rock proved to have the type of personality that it was his way or the highway, which did not mesh well with my observe-and-adjust perspective. I found his logic fascinating since nothing was black and white. He saw layers of intent in everything.

For the next two years, we received disturbing stories about Rock losing job after job due to his aggressive behavior. He locked himself in a room, chained himself to his bed at night for fear of harming people, and so on. My wife grew increasingly concerned, calling her sister often to provide wellness checks. Rock spent hours in online chat rooms talking with others about end-of-the-world events and had a string of inpatient stays in mental health units only to be released for refusing medications.

Two more years passed as my wife's family lived in Georgia and we lived in California. We took a family trip to Florida and rented a spacious Airbnb together. The first night, Rock started a conversation with me that would last the entire three days of our vacation off and on. He spoke of being "selected" as a child by a coven that chose him to be the "Black Messiah." Even though we were on vacation, I had to hear this story. He went into detail about setting the arrangement. He described multiple candidates from "G.O.D." (Guild of Doctors) that made decisions for the betterment of each region. He stated that those who were not selected were high-class citizens whose families were in an uproar and that they burned his mother to death in her home trying to find him, but he was brought into a new family to protect the future of the world.

There are narratives that make you smile or laugh immediately, and there are narratives that make you cringe and become deeply uncomfortable. But when you have heard so many stories, the narratives simply are the narratives, and the fascination is merely the telling by the narrator. Having a master's in psychology and a master's in social work, and working for many years in mental health, I knew I just had to listen respectfully and take note of things in the narrative that did not align.

I felt God had thrown this situation in my lap so I could deal with it head-on. The next morning when we were parting, I asked Rock if I could pray for him. I prayed over his life, his family, and his future. When I finished praying, Rock said nothing in response. He simply shook my hand, quickly got in his car, and drove off.

A year later, I encountered Rock again on our family trip to meet our mutual family from Georgia at the Bible Belt in Myrtle Beach. Rock was much thinner than the last time I saw him, and he appeared to avoid conversation with anyone most of the week of vacation. I noticed that our mutual in-laws for the most part avoided him. I felt compassion for him as I realized that like many undiagnosed, untreated persons, he would be written off many people's friends lists. I caught him observing me from a distance. I spoke to those around me in our family, and he just peered over his shoulder in the distance without engaging and smirked while listening to people ask me questions.

He was visibly absent when some other family members asked me to baptize them, and yet he told me in passing that I did my good deed for the day. I anointed and prayed for a family member's infected foot that day, and Rock simply watched, said nothing, and did not engage in my prayer. I knew a conversation would come; I just did not know when it would happen. The night before we were leaving, Rock sat on the couch and started sharing abstract narratives with me. They were based on bits and pieces of ancient Egyptian folklore and Jesuit constructs, and once again, his interpretation of Scripture voided the validity of the Bible.

When I challenged him respectfully, he did not become angry or rude. He just countered with another piece of history from another time period. He concluded that I was an intelligent man and that this time provided me with an opportunity to become an apprentice to his apparent greatness as a teacher. I asked him what would happen in the case of a student becoming greater than the pinnacle created for him to learn. He marveled at this question and then restated the opportunity set before me. I informed Rock that I was in harmony with the road I was on and respectfully declined. He said he respected me and my decision, shook my hand, and proceeded to invite the family to participate in a game of cards. I found the whole ordeal fascinating at best. It is instances like these, not in a setting where I expect to encounter mental health, that mental health is placed at my doorstep and makes me profoundly aware that indeed God has provided me with a desire to help people with mental health challenges, even when the person chooses not to come to Christ. The seeds were planted, and I have faith that God will prevail against Rock's will.

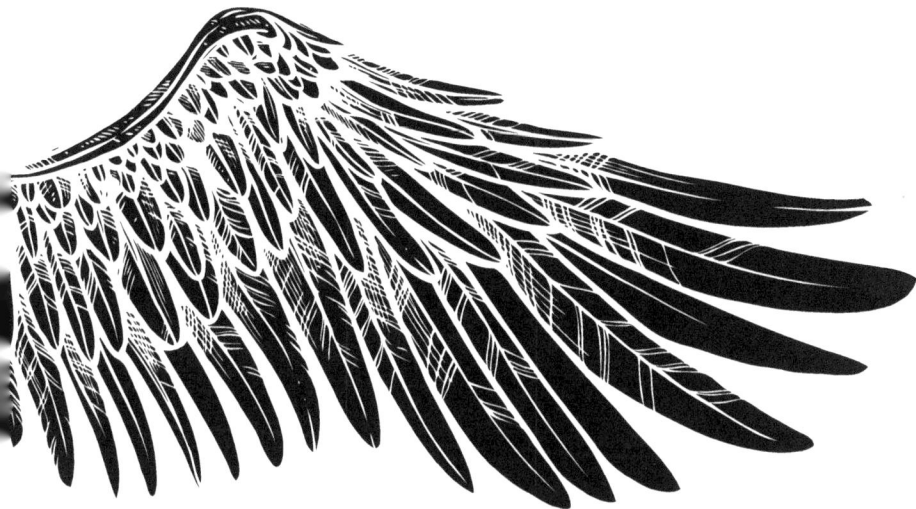

CHAPTER 9

THE OUTING

This may be your story; these may be some people you know.

*All I know is that I have seen some things that only
God could have accomplished.*

Social work can be seen through a great number of lenses. There are times when you feel as a social worker that you are on the front line of overdue, necessary changes, and then there are days you feel like no matter what impact you make, it is not enough. Sometimes you feel like you are ahead and have the recipe for any client who walks in your door, and then there are times you feel like you are the client yourself and that Groundhog Day is occurring far more often than you would like to admit.

Social work is the type of field where you are twice as likely to be cursed out for helping someone in need as you are thanked for making a difference. It is a field so misunderstood that you could fight for a degree that is much more difficult than others in mental health and still be paid wages that are competitive with a local barista's. This is not to knock the importance of a good cup of joe; this is to illustrate how seriously people take the art of mind and action.

I often think if an unhealthy mind started growing weeds out the top of their head, they would pay more attention to the upkeep. It sure would make helping people easier. I dedicated my third master's degree to God before I even started. I realized that it is God and not my own wishes that make something out of everything I have.

That surrender was the most difficult, naked, societally castrating decision ever, but once I made it, I knew it was clearly the manliest, single greatest decision ever as I stopped walking left to right trying to go straight and up and found that Christ Himself is the elevator to everything I ever wanted and needed in this life.

You do not have to take my word for it. Find out for yourself.

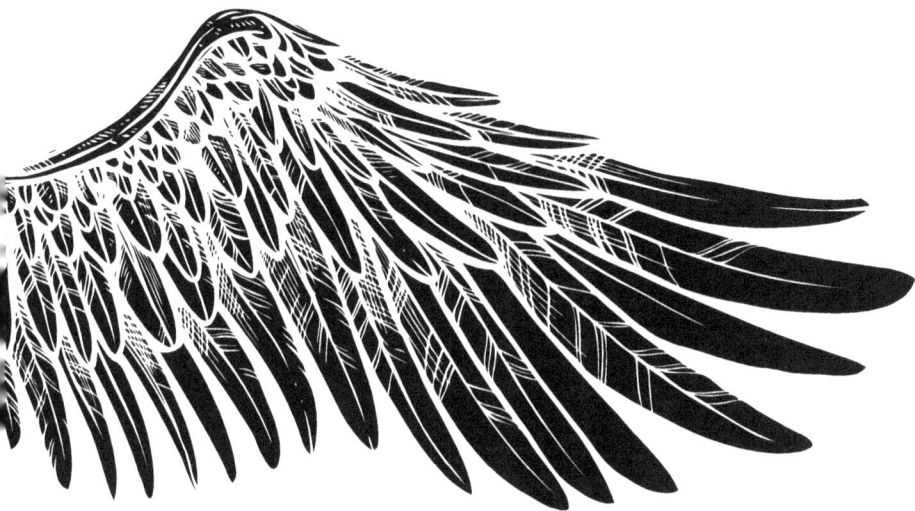

CHAPTER 10

COVID-19 AND MENTAL HEALTH

COVID-19 was strong enough to stir political unrest on any side. Gratefully, my family did not get into the hoarding toilet tissue movement. We also did not lose hours sifting conspiracy theories about who created COVID-19 and what it meant for our futures. I even laughed at a social media post claiming COVID-19 was Thanos the Destroyer resetting the universe. When COVID-19 hit the United States, I was an intern completing social work hours at a mental health unit in Newport Beach, California. The staff said there had never been a greater surge of mental health patients than during this pandemic. Depression, anxiety, suicide attempts, and suicidal ideations soared.

The staff was losing it (more than usual) as they scrambled to show clips of people collapsing all over Asia. We argued that the overpopulation of Asia was the cause of the spread and how something like the Centers for Disease Control and Prevention would be useless in many of those populations. We unanimously agreed it would never reach the United States. A month later, I had to eat those words when the dean of students emailed me and pulled the plug on all internships, effective immediately. The hospital downsized to "essential" staff for the remainder of COVID-19, and the world appeared to have gone mad.

Nothing seemed to make sense, not politically, not medically, not socially. It was as if all decisions were made by toddlers throwing darts at a wall, and that was that.

My wife, who was working in the laboratory of a major hospital, also had her faith tested by COVID-19. I kept my wife covered in prayer more than usual since her hospital was scarce on protective gear for staff and the administration was led by confusion. They were first drawing blood from COVID-19 patients with only a face covering, and then they moved to a face covering with a shield. When they understood how the virus increased, they were instructed to put on full protective gear. My wife was a hero as she worked tirelessly to help as many people as possible. I hated the circumstances; I loved the ministry it confirmed in her. I counsel many men who never get the privilege of knowing the grit in the woman they marry; I got to see it in mine.

COVID-19 hit closer to home when I got a call that Paul, my friend Michael's father, was fighting for his life against COVID-19. A month passed before we got word that he would recover. Right after that, another very close brother in Christ, a deacon in our church, and his wife who was pregnant with a miracle child contracted COVID-19 and were back in full swing merely two weeks after getting the virus. One of my wife's coworkers passed away from what was deemed "complications from conditions previous to contracting COVID-19." It was painful, it was heavy, and it was all confusing.

A Church United

During the pandemic, church and state were at war as California's Governor Gavin Newsom took a very staunch position on church restrictions, from closing the doors to opening partially, to being allowed to hold services outside, to closing again—all arguably contra-tier regulations.

At first the church appeared divided as some argued for closing to protect the people and some argued to remain open because of Hebrews 10:25.

"Not forsaking the assembling of ourselves together, as is the manner of some, but exhorting one another, and so much the more as you see the Day approaching." That Scripture was met with Scripture such as Romans 13:1–4:

Let every soul be subject to the governing authorities. For there is no authority except from God, and the authorities that exist are appointed by God. Therefore whoever resists the authority resists the ordinance of God, and those who resist will bring judgment on themselves. For rulers are not a terror to good works, but to evil. Do you want to be unafraid of the authority? Do what is good, and you will have praise from the same. For he is God's minister to you for good. But if you do evil, be afraid; for he does not bear the sword in vain; for he is God's minister, an avenger to execute wrath on him who practices evil.

Scriptures like endless thoughts ran through my head, some for closing churches, some against closing churches. I wrestled with the best approach, so I cannot fathom the weight of pastors during that time. I served during the quarantine. Our pastor was unwavering in his decision that it was our constitutional right as well as our biblical position to keep the church's doors open during this pandemic. I had to serve. I did not always have to agree, but I had to be of service. I respected that many churches provided their services online. I respected that many churches fought to stay open if it was for the right reasons. Our lead pastor took a position to keep the doors open during COVID-19, and it was the hope the community needed.

Hope. Our pastor said hope used to be found in the church during times like this and always should. He argued that the church used to be a safe haven, a sanctuary if you will. So initially, the church opened with face masks and six feet of distance, and then it progressed to open seating indoors and choosing if you wanted to sit or not or wear a mask or not. Our church never backed away from praising, worshipping, and singing for God. The church took precautions by wiping down and spraying everything in the building, but it would not compromise for mandates against our fundamental freedoms and constitutional rights.

I was a leader at a well-respected Southern California church that took a clear stand, and no member of the church became positive with COVID-19. We felt invincible. We were still shaking hands, hugging, sparingly wearing masks, and defying anything that would keep us apart. I saw COVID-19 as a faraway issue until my personal mentor, Pastor Johnny Thompson, fell ill with COVID-19. I cannot script this. This was the very same man I respected with such a high regard that I asked him to honor me by writing the foreword to this book. One of my personal heroes in the body of Christ fell ill with COVID-19. If I am honest, it seemed manageable before this "Superman" got it. I had a helpless feeling in the pit of my stomach.

A month later, I sat with Pastor Johnny and heard him speak about having convulsions and an inability to breathe. Hearing about the aches and pains of COVID-19 and how he faced death in quarantine made me fight back tears that were welling up in my spirit. I was hurt just hearing how much trouble he had simply walking from one room to another. I was hurt because he did not deserve this, not such an incredible man of God who had sacrificed so much just to love people. How could he get this horrible virus?

I never had to ask him if he got depressed or filled with anxiety or if his faith wavered. Christ was interwoven into his being, and even facing death did not scare this man. It was on that day as I sat across the table from this superhero of our time that I accepted that it was not the virus in Pastor Johnny that defined him. It was how he endured the virus, never wavering in his servitude and continuing to worship and praise God even if the situation he was in was not what he wanted or expected. Even if COVID-19 had taken his life, it would not have killed him. He was too dipped in the Holy Spirit!

I accepted that it was not the virus in Pastor Johnny that defined him. It was how he endured the virus, never wavering in his servitude and continuing to worship and praise God even if the situation he was in was not what he wanted or expected.

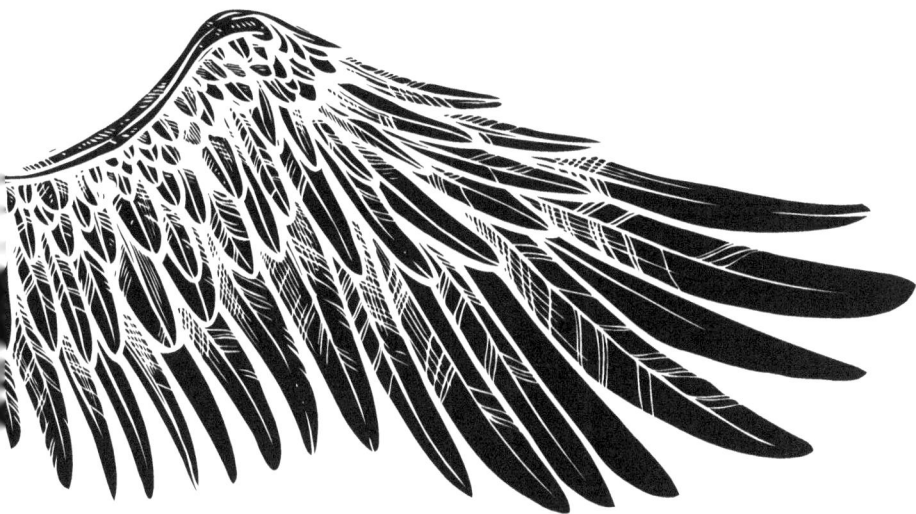

CHAPTER 11

WE ARE ALL GOING TO GET IT

We have to accept the fact that we are all going to get COVID-19.

—My former CEO

The CEO of my former employer traveled to Mexico in the middle of the pandemic to visit her spouse, knowing that he had tested positive for COVID-19. She did not divulge that she was with him until she was back and coughed and sneezed over everything in our facility for a week. I questioned her about why she would put our staff and clients at risk through exposure, and she replied, "My oldest lives in the Midwest and was one of the first to test positive. He has now had COVID-19 twice. Another one of my children has had it already, and now my husband. Antonio, we have to accept the fact that we are all going to get COVID-19."

Rebuke is what my mind thought. "The hell we all are!" is what my mouth said. Those seemingly careless, thoughtless words haunted me in following months. I left that position a month later. Four staff out of 16 fell to COVID-19, and as more of my friends and distant family members tested positive, my boss's words unfortunately played like a dreadful melody in my head.

Her words were a very real fear for me. Serving in church on Thursday nights and Sundays was the only time except in my own home that I took off my mask. It was not that I could not wear a mask in church. It was that I did not want to feel like the only person wearing a mask, and that was when new evidence emerged that wearing a mask all the time caused COVID-19 because our bodies were not creating natural immunities.

My Turn

I think it was inevitable that a few church members got COVID-19, but it did not originate from our church members. I believe it came from a crusade that used our church for a gathering of thousands of people looking to be healed from various illnesses—illnesses like COVID-19.

In January 2021, our parking lot attendants fell ill, then a few in our host team, and then outbreaks here and there left and right. We had just completed a church-wide 21-day fast, and I had a new leadership position in the church as well as a new career, which explained the headaches and nausea that typically happen when I deprive my body of food during stressors. By day three, I had constant headaches, diarrhea, and bad lower back pain, and I was urinating every half hour even when I decreased my liquid intake. I denied it in my mind, but I knew something was wrong, especially when I lost my sense of smell even before being tested for COVID-19.

I was in this drive-through of dread with my wife and four-year-old daughter, Ariel. We decided not to test my 14-year-old son, Kareem, because like many teenagers, he had not been in close contact with the family in more than a year since Xbox and PlayStation 4 had consumed 14 to 17 hours of his day. We made the mistake of providing him electronic freedom if his grades were good. Well, he ended up with great grades right before a pandemic hit that brought the school district to Zoom courses on a strict pass-or-fail contingency. We felt so bad that his first year of high school was spent online with little to no contact with his friends. We allowed him to be raised by *Call of Duty: Modern Warfare* and *Assassin's Creed Valhalla*, and of course, we had to buy him Oculus for his virtual reality friendships. It was a rough time for our son.

Back to COVID-19. It was a long line at Kaiser Permanente Irvine that day. Hazmat suits and white pop-up tents looked like a scene out of every zombie show and movie I had ever watched. I said, "This is so unrealistic." My wife scolded me for serving at church while not wearing a mask and that this was the result. I reminded her that I am a leader at church and must be about my Father's business. That did not go over well. She was right. I should have worn a mask. I cringed when I thought about it. It was just so weird with everyone not wearing a mask, none of us getting sick, and then it suddenly hitting us like a tsunami.

How humbling it was as my wife and I fell ill. My mind went to Matthew where Jesus was being tested by Satan after being baptized and told Satan in response to his advances, "You shall not tempt the LORD your God" (Matt. 4:7). We really believed we were above getting COVID-19. When the Black Plague hit eons ago, many churches remained open to prove their faith over circumstance, only to be utterly decimated. But were they? Mankind looks at the outside appearance, and God looks at the heart.

*Do we know the reasons behind remaining open as
a church? Would it have been worth it to close the
doors based on fear? The truth is that there was no
right or wrong answer.*

Like baptism by sprinkling or full immersion, it was a matter of opinion. If you closed your church doors to protect your flock, amen. If you kept your doors open to provide a haven for those desperately needing God during that time, amen.

Recall Shadrach, Meshach, and Abednego in Daniel when, in response to the decree by King Nebuchadnezzar to bow to him, they told him their God had the power to deliver them from the fiery furnace that the king threatened to throw them into. But with even deeper faith, they said, "Our God whom we serve is able to deliver us from the burning fiery furnace, and He will deliver us from your hand, O king. But if not, let it be known to you, O king, that we do not serve your gods, nor will we worship the gold image which you have set up" (Dan. 3:17–18). I have read this many times, but as I always say:

*There are times in your life when Scripture
whispers, times when Scripture appears bold, and
times when Scripture roars in your life. This time
it roared. God never needed our brazen chests and
the sound of our clanging voices like cymbals. God
wanted us to be extensions of Himself—His love,
His grace, and His mercy.*

Some postings that church members put on social media came across as arrogant and misrepresented us as a church. We love God, we love our community, we respect the differences in the body of Christ, and we do not look at those differences as a lack of faith. Paul tells us not to judge whether one believer eats or drinks and the other does not. That speaks volumes about our church conflicts today. We must have accountability to the Word of God, not a blind allegiance to popular opinion.

On January 25, 2021, I got the results that I was positive for COVID-19.

I was in self-quarantine in my home, reading the Word of God, pleading with Him to speak to me. It was the most uninterrupted time I'd had with God in years. I called on Him to use my life or take me home. I knew I had a greater purpose—loving God better, loving his flock more deeply. In the words of the time, "It is the way."

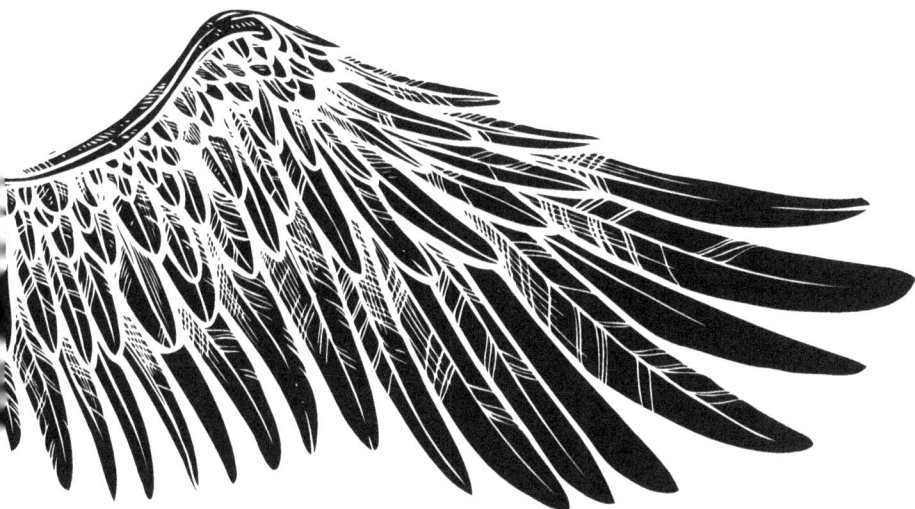

CHAPTER 12

THE YOGA-PSYCH-SURFERS OF OC

It is not uncommon for an inpatient program in Orange County to have clinical directors who have the requirements of Western medicine while holding an Eastern medicine approach to the field. The clinical portions of the entire facility were drenched in the philosophies of Buddha, Zen-type modalities, chakras, and libraries of books that covered transferring your body from one place to another using meditation. Oddly there was nothing on Christ or the God of Isaac, Abraham, and Moses.

That was not surprising since most believers know that only the truth causes conflict.

These differences can become a bridge or an altar for sacrifice, and your approach will determine your options. At that time, I was hired by the clinical director, Dr. Vigeant. She looked anything but doctoral in her presentation, which was comforting to say the least. She was wearing a mask as she ushered me into her hand-painted, turquoise office with aquatic themes, including crystal dolphins and kaleidoscope mermaids in whimsical forms.

Dr. Vigeant had lake-blue eyes and long, surfer-blond hair. Roxy was her style. She also wore these dope gold-rimmed glasses that only a legit mob boss would wear. In my more than 20 years of history in mental health, she had hands down the greatest clinical mind I had ever encountered. She could sit with a client, give them a side hug, and with precision provide them with a detailed list of what was going on in their brain, mind, and behaviors. It was masterful and beautiful to watch, and it was always done with pinpoint accuracy and a deep sense of care. Dr. Vigeant was never too proud to not take her glasses off, hold a client's hand, and shed tears with them, and for the very first time, most of them would finally begin to understand themselves in the raw. She was rightfully matched by her fiancé, Logan, who looked like a Ken doll and was an incredibly wise and enlightened man with the abilities of a therapist, yet he liked Eastern philosophies and various yoga techniques.

What Dr. Vigeant termed "organic teaching" became effective as a tool. I will not soon forget one of my clients who became furious at the amount of time we were spending outdoors creating things and the like.

Client: I'm sorry but I have to say something. Why the hell are we not learning anything with all the damn money my insurance is spending? We should be learning about addiction and overcoming mental health issues and such. This place is just weird. I have been to over 10 treatment facilities, and this is the only place that has not taught me anything.

Me (smiling): I get it. If I am hearing you right, you feel that in this setting you are not getting what you need to do well once you are discharged from the program, right?

Client: Exactly. What the hell?

Me: Okay, let me challenge that perspective. How many times have you taken substances since you have been here in our facility?

Client: Zero. There are no drugs if I wanted to, anyway.

Me: Fair enough. How many times this week did you feel like committing suicide?

Client: I have not thought of committing suicide at all this week, just thought about going to another program.

Me: You have been here three weeks, and the first week you reported having anxiety so bad that you were up at night having tremors and experiencing suicidal ideations nightly, as well as wanting drugs at least three times daily. Now you are sleeping 8–10 hours a night, have decreased anxiety and no suicidal thoughts, and you're not craving drugs. I would say that is a vast improvement with little effort needed to sustain it once you are in your own environment, right?

Client: What if doing better is just the medications?

Me: If it were just medications, then why weren't you complying with medications when you were at home? It seems simple enough, and there is nothing indicating that you cannot administer medications on your own. The truth is that you are uncomfortable with the change. I have provided nothing that you cannot do on your own at home. You can take walks in the morning, you can hike in your community, you can visit the beach as needed, you can make your own food, you can make your bed in the morning, and you can create projects around your home. I don't provide someone to stand in front of you with diagrams, charts, and traditional methods. The reason is that at home you will not have the luxury of someone standing in front of you and teaching you anything, and we as humans only retain 10–15 percent of what we hear. While away from home, struggling with mental health or addiction, I would think that number would decrease dramatically. You are now healthy enough to be away from suicidal thinking, and now you want to complain about how your life is lived.

I think subconsciously that is a win as you previously did not care, and now you want more.

Client: Crap! That just blew my mind wide open. I didn't even see it that way. It's true because I have been to all these places that do it the same way, and when I get something entirely different, I think it is not working. I get it.

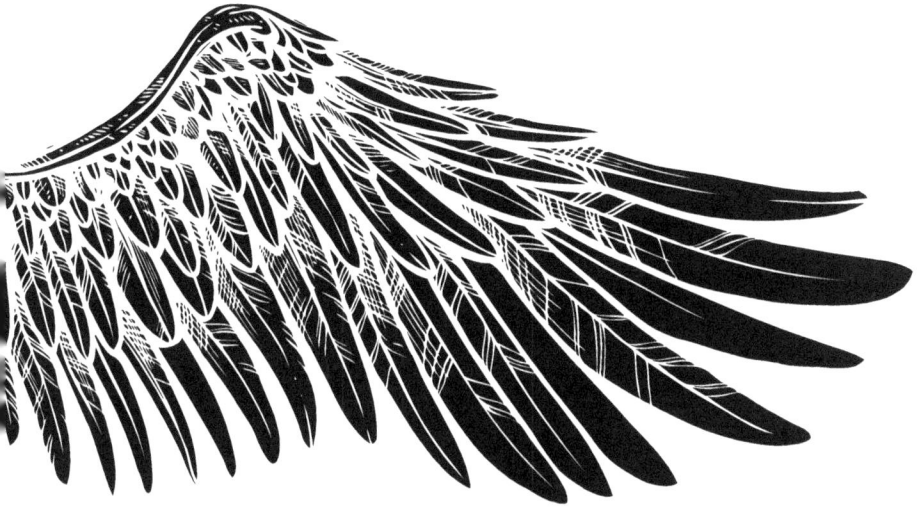

CHAPTER 13

CLINICAL CASES

Maurya It Is

Clinical diagnosis: Maurya was diagnosed with F33.2 major depressive disorder, recurrent episode, severe, F41.1 generalized anxiety disorder, F43.10 post-traumatic stress disorder, F64.0 gender dysphoria in adolescents and adults, and F60.3 borderline personality disorder.

Body Dysmorphia—Cutting

Dan was a client in a mental health facility I worked for. He was another therapist's client and steered clear of me at all costs for his first two weeks in residential care. On a random day when Dan's primary therapist was not available, Dan just waltzed into my office like we were age-old friends, sat down, and started talking to me about his life, not giving me an opportunity to object. Let me paint a picture of our first official introduction.

Dan was the shorter side of 5'5" and Caucasian. He was heavyset with big, sad brown eyes, and donned an army-style haircut. He was wearing a derogatory T-shirt of two characters flipping each other off and camo shorts with black Vans sneakers. He reminded me of that kid Sid on *Toy Story* who tried way too hard to be "bad to the bone." The clothing and haircut choices were that of a young, questionable, rebellious teen. Dan loved the spotlight on himself because Dan felt unnoticed and unwanted. That is important to note in how you approach a "Dan."

Immediately, I knew Dan suffered from a spirit of rejection.

This caused Dan's desire to be seen and heard to come across as obnoxious, simply because Dan felt if he kept talking, he would say something that people connected with.

Erik Erikson was an American German-born developmental psychologist and psychoanalyst known for creating a theory on the stages of psychosocial development. The first stage, known as trust vs. mistrust, was our focus for Dan because it is the stage he was stuck in. This stage is also known as hope and occurs during the infancy stage of 0–18 months of life. Trust vs. mistrust is the stage where a child gains a sense of trustworthiness, a sense of personal meaning, and so forth. Children develop trust in others to support their growth. In short, if they can trust the people who brought them into the world, they can trust the world. If not, they will feel the world is a hopeless and untrustworthy place. If not addressed, it is a challenge to battle as they get older.

Dan and I had one conversation, and he asked for me to become his primary therapist. As I got to know Dan, he revealed that his father was cold and absent throughout his life. He also shared that his relationship with his mother was worse because he felt his mother never loved him. When Dan was a few months old, his mother met a man who had no children and no desire to raise someone else's children. Dan shared, "My mother made the difficult decision to drop me off at my grandmother's doorstep and walk away." Dan was a master at sarcasm to soften the blows of a hard-knock life. I reminded Dan that there was no need for masks with me. It was perfectly okay to be "not okay" in my office. Dan often wiggled in his seat and didn't respond except for looking at me and giving me a half grin.

Dan cried as he lamented his mother getting pregnant twice by the man who wanted no kids and how the two sons they raised were like a brand-new family. Dan said his mother thought it was best that Dan stay away from them, but she sent Dan lots of money so she would come across as a caring parent. My objectivity was under stress, but I withheld my professionalism. Dan said his mother still talks to him, but it is like talking to a distant relative and not her own son. Dan was raised by his grandmother and called her "mother." His biological father was rarely allowed in his grandmother's home when Dan was growing up due to suspicions of his father's sexual inappropriateness with minors. Dan said there were a lot of rumors, but no one knew if they were true or not. His grandmother had strict rules for visitations, which had to remain in the living room in clear view. Dan's father insisted that he and Dan hang out in the basement during his visits to talk and watch television in private. He did that whenever Dan's grandmother was not there when he randomly showed up at the door.

On one of those occasions, Dan recalled being in the basement around 8:00 or 9:00 p.m. with his dad. He reluctantly shared that when he was on his dad's lap, his dad gave him sour-tasting orange juice while they watched cartoons. Dan fell asleep. He said he woke up to the sound of the clanky keys his father wore on his belt loops, and he was zipping up his pants. When I asked if his father often took his pants off while watching television, Dan quickly exclaimed, "No!" and then quickly stated that his dad was probably just trying to be comfortable because of all the keys, and nothing probably happened. I did not want to challenge that concept; Dan was not ready.

Two days after Dan's father left him in the basement, the grandmother told Dan that his father had been arrested for sexually assaulting a young teenage girl behind a row of high bushes as she walked home from a house party. After his grandmother handed him the newspaper, Dan read it on her front porch and crumbled to the floor. From that day on, Dan never contacted his father or vice versa. The relationship was severed.

In the field of mental health, extreme changes in appearance come from trauma at an early age. Dan had trauma from neglect and emotional and sexual abuse.

We may see the same type of presenting symptoms, yet a client's coping mechanisms will dictate the treatment modality. One of the first-impression details I left out was one of the most obvious. Dan presented with a mosaic of scar tissue that covered his entire body. Dan was a cutter. I have seen many self-harm clients in this field, but Dan was one of the most dedicated self-harm clients I had ever encountered.

Cutters become that way as a response to trauma, and cutting becomes a path out of the numbing state they are accustomed to. At times, it is a form of self-punishment for the guilt or shame they carry with them. For Dan, cutting brought attention to him. People felt sorry for him and rushed to help and give him the attention he craved. It was all eyes on Dan for a moment in time. I started praying for Dan under my breath the moment I met him. Dan made it clear to the staff that he did not want to work with a male therapist. I was intrigued because that indicated to me that his trauma probably came from a male figure. It also made me question the bond between Dan and his father and what his mental data banks recalled about that relationship.

The self-harm started to make sense. Cutting was writing the story of what was going on in Dan's life. At the time, my daughter, Ariel, was three years old, and we were watching Disney's *Moana*. In that movie, as the hero, Maui, experienced new things, a new tattoo telling his life story ended up on his skin.

Great therapy pulls up trauma from the roots.

Resurfacing deep trauma in Dan's life that he tried so desperately to avoid brought the cutting into the facility. We kept Dan from objects and provided safety contracts, 24-hour observation, rewards for not cutting, and more. Still, Dan cut. "What if the real problem was how we saw the cutting?" I thought of Maui and of the many tribes who use what we consider in America to be self-harm. Other cultures consider it a badge of honor. I decided to research that concept and put it into practice.

I asked Dan where he learned to cut himself, and after a few clearly bogus stories, he told me a story about his cousin. Jake was a few years older than Dan, and Dan's grandmother moved Jake in when Jake's mother and father split and he had nowhere else to go. Jake was described by Dan's grandmother as an angry, manipulative boy and later said she should have kept Jake away from Dan and let him go.

I probed the relationship between Dan and Jake. Dan said that one time he was changing clothes when Jake was in the room, and when he exposed his nakedness, Jake touched him, but they would not do much because Jake said Dan's body was disgusting and too fat. Dan repeatedly said that Jake verbally ridiculed and degraded him and then manipulated him into a state of control through backhanded compliments. Dan's grandmother said she believed Jake and Dan were intimate because they acted like estranged lovers. Jake was mean, and Dan pined for Jake's approval. Jake was a narcissist, a difficult pairing for anyone, especially someone with low self-esteem. Dan was attracted to Jake like a magnet to a fridge, but narcissists cannot be pleased, and Dan was ill-equipped for a "Jake."

Grandma said she just did not have room under one roof to keep Dan from Jake's venom. Dan became uncomfortable when questions of possible intimacy came up. Dan also reported that Jake was his gateway to cutting. When Jake thought about his mother and father fighting, he cut himself so one day his parents would see all his cuts and know how their fighting had affected him. He did it in hopes that they would feel sorry for him and his sacrifice would be the key to putting his family back together. Jake had to be the hero—textbook narcissism.

Dan was easy prey. Dan bought into the ideal and began to cut his story on his body. He used self-harm to escape trauma but also to express his shame, his guilt, and his frustrations. The problem was that Jake kept his cutting light and in places beneath the naked eye, mostly because in his mind, everything was everyone else's fault. Dan, on the other hand, remained in a constant state of trauma, depression, guilt, shame, and frustration, so the cutting increased. Dan used any sharp object—broken mirrors, razors, nails, hairpins, hangers, his own fingernails that he bit off and rubbed back and forth in his skin to cause marks, and when all else was unavailable, he bit himself until he bled.

When Dan spoke about the first time he cut himself, he mimicked the behavior of a first-time heroin addict. He talked about the naughtiness of it as he sat in a graveyard with Jake. He talked about the rush as the blood went trickling down his wrists. As he spoke, my mind was already trying to think of various strategies and coping alternatives to cutting. Shortly after Jake taught Dan how to cut, Jake's parents got back together and took him away from Dan, who would later admit that it was best for his life. At that point, Dan was already doing anything to please Jake and keep Jake from being angry at him.

Because Dan did not know it was best for him at the time, he cut even more because he felt abandoned yet again. When Dan talked about this period of his life, he was more emotional than he had ever been, and it struck a chord with me. I wanted to hug Dan and let him know he would be okay, but professionally, I had to help Dan feel all the emotions he had worked so hard to avoid. He had to know that emotions would not destroy him. Letting him feel them all provided Dan with the certainty that those emotions would not kill him. They were simply emotions he gave power to. The session that really hit home for Dan was when I told him to sit still and pay attention.

Face every emotion that comes to you. Address each by name, reframe them from a position of power, and repurpose any negative thoughts toward those emotions from a noose around your neck into a badge of honor.

Dan said those words were a turning point in his life. He responded, "Hold every thought in captivity." It was what I had said in every one of our sessions. Dan gave me a puzzled look and then asked, "Mr. Anderson, do you read the Bible? Because I heard that before." That might have been the first smile he ever gave me, and I decided the required professional response was inadequate for the necessity of his inquiry. "Yes, I am not just a hearer but a doer of the

Word." Dan smiled back and told me he knew it because I worded things like what he used to hear in church. I told him I never heard him talk about going to church and reminded him that he stated on his initial assessment that he had no religion or spiritual support.

During the time he lived with his grandmother, a friend invited him to church and sometimes read the Bible to him. Dan had a very skewed understanding of the Bible. He often misquoted and misinterpreted Scripture based on his personal beliefs. In Dan's mind, God was an all-powerful bully sitting high on a throne, throwing condemnation at us from a world away. That was also why Dan carried all his guilt and shame as if he were in purgatory for crimes. Together through the reframing of his experiences, Dan realized he did not deserve the abandonment and traumas. He ultimately came to the conclusion that his wounds were unique and that God loved him and would use his story as a testimony to reach many others just like him.

Over the next few weeks, I worked with Dan. The sessions shifted from learning to cope with what had already happened to what the Bible meant for Dan's future. Dan ended up asking for a Bible, and administration would have a war about that. Apparently, yoga, chakras, guided meditation, burning sage, hanging crystals, burning incense, and books on transporting your soul from one place to another were all acceptable. But the name of Jesus and the power of His blood were where they drew the line.

A few weeks went by, and Dan asked to pray with me. I obliged and asked, "Who does God know you as?" I showed him a skit on YouTube by a group called Lifehouse. It was called "Broken." It depicted a young woman born dancing with Jesus and how she was oblivious to the world in a dance with Jesus before Satan and the temptations of the world entered her life and tried to destroy her. The climax of the skit was when the girl had enough and was holding a gun to her head. Suddenly she remembered she is a child of God and started fighting to be in a relationship with Christ. The whole time, Christ was present, but Christ never put the girl in that prodigal situation. It was by her free will that she walked in and by her free will that she could call upon His name and He would fight her battles. Dan wanted to see it twice. Then he smiled a gigantic smile that reached ear to ear and replied, "Jesus was calling to her from a distance. He never left her. He was waiting for her to want Him back." Then the girl said, "That is my story."

Dan said, "If we are going to pray, God knows me as Maurya." In a little office in Southern California, thousands of miles from her Chicago home, 24 years after her birth, Maurya finally felt enough to be herself. The spirit of God filled the room, and I could see her walls coming down in the spiritual realm. I asked Maurya if we could pray. She reached her hands across the table into mine and asked Christ into her heart that moment. I would love to say that the cutting stopped immediately, but it did not. Maurya continued over the next month to cut from time to time and struggle, but she was struggling forward. The cutting would decrease, and she would vow to stop.

Once the seed is planted, we must trust that God has
a plan to continue the growth.

Through a spiritual lens, Maurya was suffering from generational curses and demonic oppression. Maurya was led to believe all the lies that were constantly fed to her and was born with open portals through initial abandonment and rejection. Her cutting and torment reminded me of the story in Mark 5.

> *Then they came to the other side of the sea, to the*
> *country of the Gadarenes. And when He had come*
> *out of the boat, immediately there met Him out of*
> *the tombs a man with an unclean spirit, who had his*
> *dwelling among the tombs; and no one could bind*

him, not even with chains, because he had often been bound with shackles and chains. And the chains had been pulled apart by him, and the shackles broken in pieces; neither could anyone tame him. And always, night and day, he was in the mountains and in the tombs, crying out and cutting himself with stones.

When he saw Jesus from afar, he ran and worshiped Him. And he cried out with a loud voice and said, "What have I to do with You, Jesus, Son of the Most High God? I implore You by God that You do not torment me."

For He said to him, "Come out of the man, unclean spirit!" Then He asked him, "What is your name?"

—Mark 5:1–9

This is from a book written thousands of years ago that applies to what we deal with today. "Assuredly, I say to you, whatever you bind on earth will be bound in heaven, and whatever you loose on earth will be loosed in heaven" (Matt. 18:18).

This verse is power, and we should be praying about every situation. We should never cease praying since each prayer is one prayer closer to a miracle being unleashed in our lives.

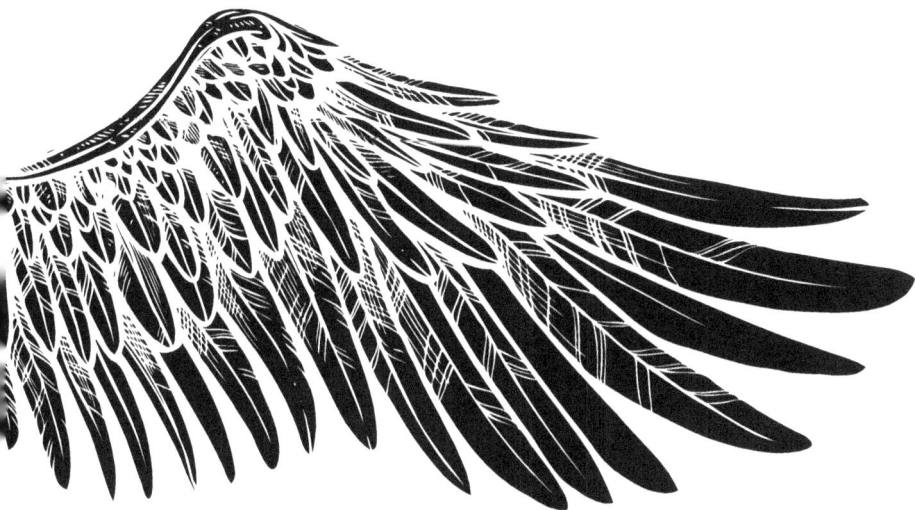

CHAPTER 14

VIN "RACER" NORWAY

F33.2 Major depressive disorder, recurrent episode, severe
F41.1 Generalized anxiety disorder
G31.84 Mild neurocognitive disorder due to traumatic brain injury
F41.0 Panic disorder
F51.01 Insomnia disorder
Pseudobulbar effect

Vin stood out to me immediately because he presented like Orange County royalty. He was middle-aged and had deep, thinking man's features. He dressed like he was sponsored by REI. Vin was a high-profile client who was a professional Formula 1 race car driver. His presenting issue was that he was sent to me from a mental health hospital after being stabilized from a suicide attempt three days prior. Vin had launched his car off a cliff along Pacific Coast Highway to end it all. The question was why? On paper it didn't make sense. Vin had achieved greatness. He had money, a beautiful wife, and five children, and the three girls all looked like mini beauty pageant winners. The two boys looked exactly like Vin but with less eyebrows.

I jumped on performing Vin's bio-psych assessment, a standard tool used when taking in a new client. It provides the therapist everything needed to create a functional treatment plan. Of course, that is if the therapist works for an organization that uses golden threads and useful treatment plans so clinical staff can work like a clinical staff should. Vin could not sit down to save his life. He walked around the room restlessly in a circle, brushing his hand against the top of his chair in a ritualistic manner each time he walked by it. Since moving the chair slightly every lap got him to stop, I was able to rule out obsessive compulsive disorder.

According to Vin, he hated his life and was too embarrassed to face how humiliating it was to be in that position. He had been married for 10 years to a woman he claimed he never loved. I asked Vin to elaborate, and he said he stole his wife from another man when she and her husband at the time were visiting from Norway on vacation. He said she was beautiful, and he could not stop flirting with her. He convinced her to leave the man she was married to and come to America. They now had five children together, but he said he was haunted by the truth that he was a liar. He then stated that if his friends knew, they would no longer like him because his wife, Sasha, was so perfect, and no one would believe he did not love her for as long as he had faked it. He peered out the window every time a car rolled by, thinking his friends or the police were coming to get him. I could not even respond before Vin blurted out, "And if the police knew I have lied this long about not loving my wife, I would be arrested!"

I forgot I was in a mental health facility and responded, "If they arrested men for not being in love with their wives, I think Orange County would have a lot of fresh real estate." Vin stared at me blankly, and I immediately followed up. "Vin, why would the police be concerned whether you loved your wife or not?"

Vin said it was the deception that would do him in.

Everything outside of delusions and his constant pacing indicated that he was normal. It was the amount of outward "normalcy" that made his absurd notion that he was in trouble for not loving his wife seem like he could be joking, even to a therapist. But Vin was dead serious about it. I knew this was true a few days into the sessions because in his current state, Vin could not tell a joke to save his life.

Vin was quiet, isolative, reserved, anxious, and extremely bored. These were all indications that he was going to be a handful, and the first few days were a lot of rapport building and going through the motions. During an early group I ran, without mentioning a specific Scripture, I said these words: "Do unto others as you would have them do unto you." As I was saying it, Vin was mouthing the words. I carried on with the rest of the group without addressing what he had done. I could not help but smile because I knew I found just what I needed to move mountains in Vin's psyche.

The following session we talked about his upbringing in Sweden and his faith. Vin is a Christian, and his family are long-time members of a megachurch in Orange County. He was the first client I encountered at that facility who claimed faith and brought his own Bible with him, which he read nightly. The next few weeks we went over the books of Ephesians and Proverbs. It was Christmas time, the perfect timing in Vin's life since he had to watch family traditions through Zoom and witness his wife and children baking cookies, going shopping, and attending events without him. I asked him how he felt, and he said, "I really miss my family," and then he went into detail about everything he was missing out on.

A major turning point in our work together was while we were on a walk in San Clemente. Vin and I were walking along the pier when he started scanning the area as if he were replaying memories in his head. At the end of the pier was a large Christmas tree that Vin gazed at for a while. I walked up to him and said, "You are thinking about your wife a lot today, aren't you?" Vin was surprised that I picked up on that so easily. I was not as surprised; it was written all over his face. He was hit so hard by memories of his wife that he looked puzzled. The warmth was contradictory to the anti-love campaign he had been spewing.

I liken it to the end of The Grinch *when he is standing there realizing he loved what he pretended to hate his entire life.*

Shortly after, we had a family session with his wife, and I took a gamble and asked Vin why he kept staring at his wife when she spoke. I had no idea what would come out of his mouth, and I prayed under my breath. Vin looked at her, then at me, and said, "I just can't believe how beautiful she is and how much I have put her through." She cried, and I left the rest of the session in their hands. I was rewarded for my boldness and went in again after she left. I told him he was an incredible racer and achieved much in his life, and now he had lost his zest because he had nothing to chase. He had the perfect life, which for some men is the worst thing that can happen because they plateau.

Vin sat on the edge of his seat while I spoke. His eyebrows arched up as he thought of what was left for him to accomplish.

He had done everything racing had to offer, from Norway to the big screens of Hollywood. Vin was used to hard work and being driven. Now that he had it all, he was bored. There was no carrot dangling in from him. He needed another challenge. Vin had to race. His identity was being "the Guy." My work was getting Vin to recall what he loved most about life.

Two weeks later, Vin invited me to pray over his home.

He wanted to feel the fresh start from God. He wanted his wife to feel the presence of God like we had felt in our sessions.

His wife greeted me at the door and told me she had been praying for him to encounter a man of great faith in order to change his life. I told her all praises go to God and that I am blessed to be in the position to hear God's voice. I had them hold hands while I prayed over them. Then we went from room to room praying Psalm 91, dispatching angels, breaking generational curses, allowing the Holy Spirit to flow, and casting out any demonic forces.

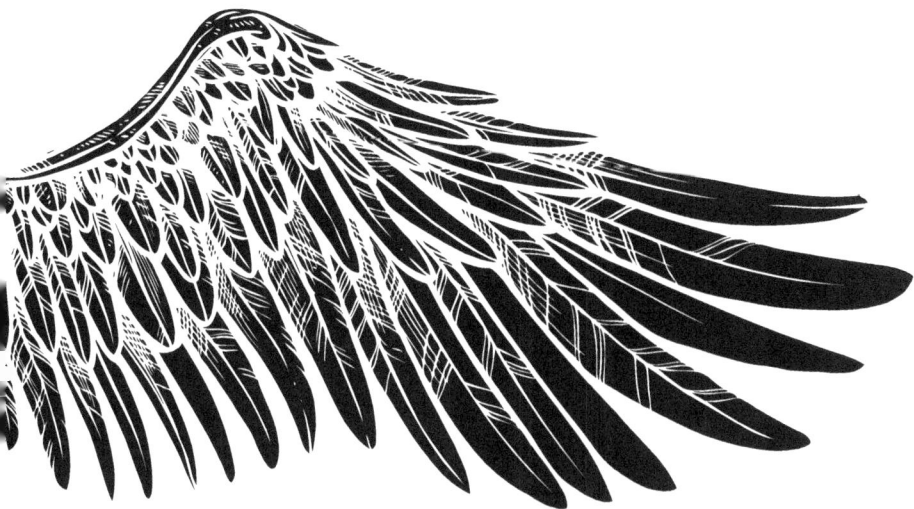

CHAPTER 15

AN EMPATH NAMED ANGEL

Angel is the only case study on this list who was not a client. Angel was a peer. She is a single, Caucasian Native American in her mid-30s who looks like Dorothy from the *The Wizard of Oz*. She is the girl next door and a single mom of four kids. If you were to look up *empath*, *genuineness*, and *warmth* in the dictionary, you would find Angel. She is the ultimate busybody. You must stretch and eat your Wheaties before you work a shift with her. I envied her incredible nonstop, self-charge battery until I got to know her on a deeper level. Angel's empathy and never-stop attitude came at a high price. She could just as likely be an enforcer in a roller derby as the belle of an extravagant ball.

Angel was dedicated to the well-being of the organization. She worked without hesitation whenever there was a need—rain, sleet, or snow. She fulfilled nursing needs and counseling needs, facilitated group needs, fixed things around the house, and purchased whatever needed to be purchased. She was like putty you could fill any hole with. Like putty, she was stuck from wall to wall so often that her sacrifices were often disregarded as just Angel being Angel.

What was worse is that Angel used her own money regardless if she was reimbursed or not. She never complained and was always loyal no matter how tough things got. She did not know how to quit. She rode the waves into an abyss and hoped for a tunnel on the other side. I saw all these as admirable qualities until I started hearing her heart through the Spirit.

On the outside, Angel was the greatest employee you ever met. But beneath the smile she always learned to wear, she was literally imploding.

Externally she was always present; internally, she was a compilation of pinpricks, deep tears, and scar tissue on the heart—a faintly beating heart struggling to keep life coursing through her veins. She appeared to have just what it took to have one foot in front of the other.

Many times, I had to avoid Angel to complete my work. I wanted to save Angel, which is my go-to behavior after my Street Sally experience as a child in San Francisco. It was difficult to see her going through such difficult times in her life and feel helpless. I heard tidbits of what her life was like, which led us into deep discussions. We increasingly ended up working side by side. As I got to know Angel more, she opened up about her late-husband's passing. They were motorcycle enthusiasts, and one day on a ride, he was under the influence and a costly miscalculation cost him his life and the devastation of Angel holding him for six hours as he passed away. This event was extreme trauma for Angel since they were on the brink of becoming a power couple and finally achieving some long-term goals they had set.

Later, the entire story revealed just how deep that was for Angel who was, even in those days, barely keeping it together since her marriage had taken a heavy toll with too many empty promises and unwarranted patience to only end up with fool's gold time after time. She loved her husband, even for all the things he was not, for the many times he recklessly hurt himself, hurt her, disappointed the children, and left her with the remnants. Yet Angel believed in for better or for worse and til death do us part, and she was a hopeless romantic who would do whatever it took to have a fairy-tale ending.

What was amazing about Angel is that she was not concerned with all the men who found her attractive or desired her. She wanted to be kept by one good man who could love her and her kids and keep a commitment. This, too, would prove difficult since the very next man who professed to want a future with Angel took his own life shortly after proposing to her. Angel was left shattered, finding his body hanging in the bathroom. She was hurt and confused and attempted to hide her own emotions while consoling his two young daughters he left behind.

On one occasion when we were discussing why she was not out there making friends and meeting new people, tears welled up in her eyes, and she exclaimed, "I just want someone who will love me and not die!" It was simple, it was devastating, and it was powerful, and all I could do was hug her.

One day Angel will know her worth beyond her work. I long for that day that she will not look for an occupation to keep her.

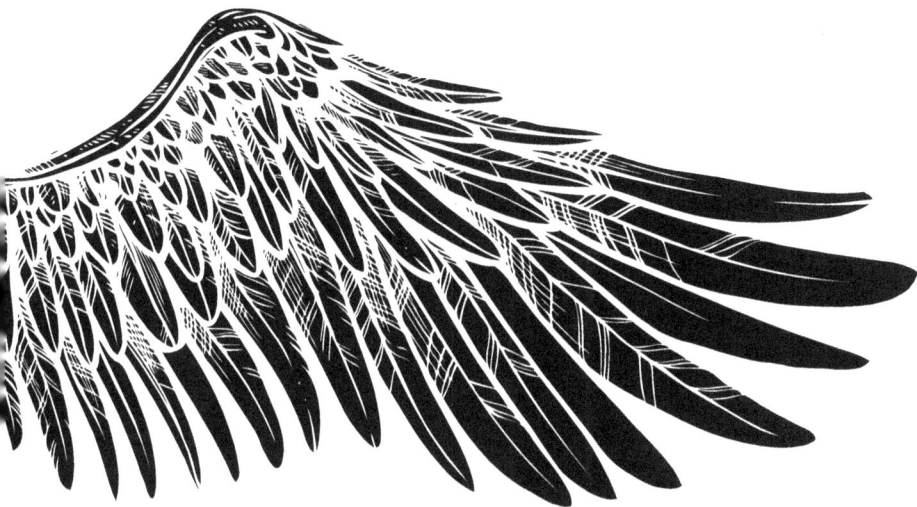

CHAPTER 16

THE FINAL CHAPTER

Satan used mental illness in the form of torment, depression, strife, anger, bitterness, and jealousy, all passed down to Adam and Eve's son Cain who killed his brother, Abel. Psychological terms such as "mental illness" are what we now use to describe what was termed back then by the Greeks *daimonion*, which translates to "devil' or "demonic." It was used to describe people who were considered possessed. That left us open to any and every attack of the devil's schemes.

That is, until God sent His Son Jesus to be the perfect and spotless lamb to die for our sins on the cross. Jesus took every sin upon His person and not only died but rose on the third day to conquer sin and bridge the gap between God and mankind. And the only thing we must do to gain purpose in this life is believe and receive that truth.

*It seems too good to be true, too easy a price for
all the sins we recall committing against God, yet
imagine that it only took a bite of a forbidden fruit
to ruin paradise, and it takes faith the size of a mere
mustard seed to move mountains.*

Christ's death was for your gain, and His sacrifice was for your endless future and eternity when people will return to a right standing with God. All you must do is accept this golden ticket.

*If God left the 99 for the one, imagine that you alone
are worth Him dying for.*

Authority was restored to mankind through Christ. We have a choice to give it back to Satan or tap into that authority. How do we exercise this authority? We do it through our spoken Word. The power of life and death are in the spoken Word. "Death and life are in the power of the tongue, and those who love it will eat its fruit" (Prov. 18:21). Matthew 10:8 tells us, "Heal the sick, cleanse the lepers, raise the dead, cast out demons. Freely you have received, freely give." In the Bible we never read about Jesus getting on his knees and praying, "God, if it be your will, please heal this man of the demons that are possessing him."

Jesus spoke with authority, commanding demons to flee and people to be healed from afflictions. Luke 10:17 states, "Then the seventy returned with joy, saying, 'Lord, even the demons are subject to us in Your name.'" They had swagger because the name of Jesus gave them power. Mark 13:34 reminds us that we have the same authority and swagger from Christ that they had. "It is like a man going to a far country, who left his house and gave authority to his servants, and to each his work, and commanded the doorkeeper to watch."

In faith and in the name of Jesus, command with authority in His power and not your own. All demons, sickness, and warfare are subject to the power of Christ and must flee now! Do not plead with demons, do not beg, do not ask, do not be polite. Be bold with authority like the woman who knew without a question or a doubt that if she could just get through the crowd enough to touch the hem of Jesus's garment, she would be healed.

Be bold in knowing that the assignment of these demons is to do their part to steal, kill, and destroy the Kingdom of God.

You have the weapon of all weapons at your disposal when you are a child of God and claim the blood of Jesus over your enemies and into your life.

You are meant to be courageous! This short life on earth is but a vapor in the wind and nothing compared to eternity in the new, flawless body and mind we will have.

REFERENCES

Hamer, D. (2005). *The God Gene: How Faith Is Hardwired into Our Genes.* Anchor Books.

Silveira, L. A. (2008). "Experimenting with Spirituality: Analyzing *The God Gene* in a Nonmajors Laboratory Course." *CBE Life Sciences Education,* 7(1), 132–145.

Wade, N. (2009, November 14). "The Evolution of the God Gene." *The New York Times.*

ABOUT THE AUTHOR

ANTONIO ANDERSON has close to 20 years of experience in the mental health field and has been a licensed minister for six years. He provides therapy, counseling, life coaching, and public speaking in Los Angeles and Orange County where he resides with his beautiful wife, Adriana, his aunt Angelica, and his two children, Kareem and Ariel. Antonio holds a bachelor of science in psychology from Long Beach State University, where he was a scholar-athlete playing rugby. He has a master's degree in general psychology from Grand Canyon University, an earned master's in clinical psychology from Capella University, and a master's in social work from Walden University.

www.ingramcontent.com/pod-product-compliance
Lightning Source LLC
Chambersburg PA
CBHW071232290326
41931CB00037B/2679